Henry Horne

Essays concerning iron and steel:

The first, containing observations on American sand-iron

Henry Horne

Essays concerning iron and steel:
The first, containing observations on American sand-iron

ISBN/EAN: 9783348015592

Printed in Europe, USA, Canada, Australia, Japan

Cover: Foto ©ninafisch / pixelio.de

More available books at **www.hansebooks.com**

ESSAYS

CONCERNING

IRON and STEEL:

THE FIRST,

Containing OBSERVATIONS on
AMERICAN SAND-IRON:

THE SECOND,

OBSERVATIONS, founded on Experiments,
on Common IRON-ORE, with the Method
of reducing it firſt into PIG or SOW-METAL,
and then into BAR-IRON; on the Sort of
Iron proper to be converted into good STEEL,
and the Method of refining that Bar-Steel
by Fuſion, ſo as to render it fit for the
more curious Purpoſes: With an Account
of Mr. REAUMUR's Method of ſoftening
Caſt-Iron;

AND

AN APPENDIX,

Diſcovering a more perfeﬅ Method of Charring
PIT-COAL, ſo as to render it a proper Succedaneum for charred WOOD-COAL.

By HENRY HORNE.

LONDON:
Printed for T. CADELL, in the Strand.
M.DCC.LXXIII.

At thefe words, p 17. [I fhall not fail communicating them to you] put an afterifm, and add the following note :

The phænomenon here referred to is, that, whereas I expected it would turn out hard pigmetal, it in fact turned out tolerably malleable fteel; which was the cafe alfo in various trials upon all kinds of mine-ftone. But concerning this matter I need fay no more in this place, as it is fufficiently confidered in the Second Effay; except only juft to remark the difference, which muft of neceffity happen between an experiment made upon a fmall quantity of ore in a crucible, where the external air can have no admiffion, and that made in a large fmelting-furnace by the violent blaft of an enormous pair of bellows. In the former cafe, the efficacy of the charcaol, mixed up along with the ore, is difpenfed in a flow and nearly infenfible manner; whereas in the latter, both the ore and the coal are almoft inftantly torn to pieces, and the falt and fulphur before locked up in the charcoal are as fpeedily fet at liberty, and powerfully excited to execute their office. So that in the latter cafe, it is not at all furprizing, that the metal fhould be much harder and more fragile, than in the former; but in both cafes, it is extremely evident, that the ferrugineous atoms are fairly converted into fteel.

OBSERVATIONS

ON

AMERICAN SAND-IRON.

In a LETTER to

The late Mr. JOHN ELLICOT,
F. R. S.

Read at the ROYAL SOCIETY,
March 3, 1763.

B

OBSERVATIONS

ON

AMERICAN SAND-IRON.

To Mr. JOHN ELLICOT.

SIR,

AS the affair of the rich American
Iron Ore, commonly known by the
name of the Virginia black sand, has of
late not only engaged the conversation of
many of the Virtuosi, but has been taken
very particular notice of by the Society
for the encouragement of arts and manufactures; I thought myself obliged,
for many reasons, to lay before you what-

ever

ever has come to my knowledge relating to this difcovery, either from my own experiments, or from the information of others. And I engage in this fervice with the greater pleafure, as I look upon it to be one of the moft interefting dif-coveries, with regard to this ufeful metal, that has come to our knowledge for fome ages, and, if rightly conducted, may prove of infinite fervice to us in this part of the world, as well as to the inhabitants of our colonies, where (as it has been fuppofed, though without fufficient foundation) this difcovery was firft made.

Without any farther preface or apology, permit me to remind you, that, in a converfation which formerly paffed between us upon this fubject, I acquainted you, that, about twenty years fince, I

7   was

was engaged in making a variety of experiments upon the nature of Iron Ores, and Steel; and that I then made a very particular enquiry into the nature of this black fand, and, in the courfe of thefe experiments, feveral very interefting phenomena difcovered themfelves, which, as they might be of great fervice to the world in general, and more efpecially to fuch as are concerned in fmelting of the iron from the ore, I had thoughts of communicating to the public; but, as my bufinefs will not permit me to go through the whole at prefent, I fhall confine myfelf to what relates to the black fand.

I procured, from Mr. Adams the Virginia merchant, a fufficient quantity of the fand, and, in order to eftimate its

com-

comparative weight with that of iron ore,
I procured fome of the richeft ore I could
get, which having reduced to powder, I
filled an ordinary tea-cup with it. I afterwards filled the fame cup with fome
of the fand, and upon comparing the
weights with each other, I found that
the weight of the fand was to that of the
ore as 3 to 2; and having taken notice
how readily the fand was attracted by the
magnet, I was convinced that the fand
muft certainly contain a very confiderable
quantity of Iron, and therefore determined
to make trial of it. I was however, for
fome time, interrupted in my defign, by
information I received from a friend,
that fuch an enquiry had been made
many years before, by a member of the
Royal Society, and a gentleman of efteem
as a chemift, but without fuccefs; and

that

that the experiments were publifhed in the 2d vol. of Lowthorp's Abridgment of the Philofophical Tranfactions. As this account is very fhort as well as curious, I fhall take the liberty to give it you entire, with fome few remarks upon it.

" A black fhining fand from Virginia examined by Dr. All. Moulen.

A fmall vial filled with ordinary white fand, and containing only ʒ i. gr. xi. being filled with the Virginia fand, was found to contain ʒij. ϶ij. gr. i.

This fand did apply to the magnet both before and after calcination; but the latter did apply better to it than the former.

A parcel

A parcel of this fand, mixed and calcined with powdered charcoal, and kept
in a melting furnace for about an hour,
yielded no regulus : but applied more
vigoroufly to the Loadftone than either
of the former.

I fluxed a parcel of this fand with fixed
nitre, in a melting furnace, for above
an hour; but could obtain no regulus;
nor any fubftance that would apply to
the magnet, except a thin cruft that
ftuck firmly to a piece of charcoal that
dropt into the crucible when the matter
was in fufion.

I fluxed it alfo with falt-petre and
powdered charcoal, dropping pieces of
charcoal afterwards into the crucible. It
continued about half an hour in the
melting

melting furnace in fufion, and that without producing a regulus, or a fubftance
that would apply to the magnet, excepting only what ftuck to the charcoal
as in the former experiment.

I fluxed another parcel of it with falt-
petre and flower of brimftone, without
being able to procure any regulus.

I poured good fpirit of falt on a parcel
of this fand, but could obferve no luĉta-
tion thereby produced.

I poured fpirit of nitre, both ftrong
and weakened with water, on parcels of
the fame fand, without being able to difcover any conflict.

B 5　　　　I poured

I poured fingle aqua fortis upon another parcel of it, without being able to perceive any ebullition worth noting.

I ufed alfo double aqua fortis upon another parcel of it, which, for ought I could difcover, had no more effect on it than the former.

I poured fome aqua regia on a parcel of it, without difcovering any fenfible effect. I poured good oil of vitriol upon another parcel of this fand; but feeing no bubbles thereby produced, I weakened the oil with water, but without any vifible effect.

I repeated all the former experiments with the menftruums upon this fand after calcination per fe in a crucible, but could
fcarce

scarce obferve a bubble produced by any of them.

I poured fome of each of the liquors upon parcels of the powder of this fand calcined, without any fuccefs.

Note, That I made thefe experiments both in the cold, and upon a fand furnace. So that to me there feems to be but little wanting to difcover any metal known to us, if it contained any fuch: for there is no metal nor ore that fome of thefe men-ftruums will not work on.

I powdered a fragment of a loadftone, and poured fome of thefe menftruums upon it, without being able to find that they in the leaft preyed upon it, any more than they did upon the fand.

I poured

I poured some of the aforementioned menstruums upon ordinary sand taken out of a sand furnace, where it must have suffered some calcination; but could find no more bubbles produced thereby, than what might rationally be supposed to be produced from lime, and other dirt mixed with the sand."

Having thoroughly considered these experiments, they appeared to me far from being decisive, and that if the Doctor had placed more confidence in the power of the magnet, and less in his menstruums, he would rather have concluded that there might be some forts of iron ore which his menstruums would not touch in the moist way, nor any regulus be produced from them in the dry, as he made use of them, which yet might,

under

under fome other hands, be fubdued, by more apt and powerful methods than any which at that time he was acquainted with.

However I apprehended I might fairly draw this conclufion from his experiments, viz. that the fand was not altogether and fimply iron, but that it was ftrongly united with a very ftubborn, fixed, and permanent earth, which could not be feparated from it without fome extraordinary, as well as powerful means; but I could not think this a fufficient objection to the profecution of an experiment, which, if it fucceeded, might be attended with very happy confequences. Proceeding therefore upon this fuppofition, I mixt up about 8 or 9 ounces of the fand, with a proportional quantity of

a ftrong

a ſtrong corroſive flux, which I put together in a crucible, and committed it to
a very ſtrong fire in an excellent wind-
furnace, where I kept it for between two
and three hours, hoping by this means to
have anſwered the intended purpoſe; but
I confeſs I was not a little ſurpriſed, that,
after the crucible was taken from the
fire, I could not find one ſingle grain of
metal in the remaining contents.

This diſappointment greatly puzzled
me, till having thoroughly examined into
the unexpected event, without being able
to diſcover any reaſon ſufficient to incline
me to recede from my former opinion,
as to the component parts of the ſand, I
concluded that the flux might poſſibly
be a very improper one; for though it
might have effected the intended ſepara-
tion,

tion, yet it might at the fame time be fufficiently powerful to divide the particles of the metal, when feparated, fo very minutely, as to be capable of fubliming and carrying them off imperceptibly: And finding the contents greatly diminifhed, fo that the quantity remaining bore but a fmall proportion to that which was firft put into the crucible, I concluded that this muft really have been the cafe, and that fome very different method muft be purfued in order to produce the defired effects. I immediately determined to make a fecond trial, in which I proceeded in the following manner. I took the fame quantity of fand made ufe of in the former experiment; and firft I fpread it, without any addition to it, upon an iron plate over a ftrong fire, where I gave it a very

powerful

powerful torrification (or roafting), to try if, by that means, I could not relax, and loofen the component parts to fuch a degree, as to make the feparation and reduction of the metal more eafy, when I fhould bring it into the furnace. When I had fo done, I mixed it up with a flux of a very peculiar, but gentle nature, which I had before made ufe of for other purpofes with great fuccefs, and committed it (as in the former experiment) to the furnace, where I urged it by a very ftrong fire for about three hours, and upon taking it out, I found the event anfwerable to my moft fanguine expectations: for in the bottom of the crucible I found, as near as I can remember, rather more than half of the fand I put into the crucible reduced to a very fine malleable metal.

In

In this very agreeable experiment I met with a very furprizing phænomenon, which, as I am not at prefent able to determine whether it was only cafual, or what would always happen in the like experiments, you will excufe my divulging at prefent, efpecially as you, Sir, by furnifhing me with a frefh parcel of the fand, have enabled me to make fome farther trials; which I fhall embrace the firft opportunity of doing; and fhould I be fo happy as to confirm what I then obferved, or to make any farther difcoveries deferving your notice, I fhall not fail communicating them to you.

Being fully convinced, by the experiment, that the fand was a very rich iron ore, I acquainted fome of my friends with it, who being largely engaged in

trade

trade to thofe parts of our American colonies, where I was informed this fand
was to be eafily procured, and in very
large quantities, I was in great hopes an
account of this nature would have inclined fome of the gentlemen in that part
of the world, to have profecuted fo ufeful
a difcovery in a larger way; and I own I
have often wondered, that an affair of
fuch confequence fhould have lain dor-
mant for fo many years.

However I was a few months fince
pleafingly furprifed, to find in the hands
of my very ingenious friend Mr. Peter
Collinfon, not only a pamphlet, but likewife a letter upon the fubject addreffed to
the Society for encouraging of arts and
manufactures, by one Mr. G. Elliot, who
relates, that, though previous to his attempt

tempt of making iron from this fand, he met with nothing but what was dif-couraging from the moft fkilful perfons to whom he propofed his defign, yet that he had fuch a perfuafion in his own mind of the practicability of the thing, that he could not reft till he had made a trial, and the event proved encouraging much beyond his expectations, infomuch that he could fcarcely believe the trial had been fairly made, till a fecond trial evinced with certainty, that eighty-three pounds of the fand would produce a barr of excellent iron weighing fifty pounds: a prodigious yield indeed, and far be-yond what I have ever heard of from the richeft common ores that are any where to be found; moft of the ores I have ever met with or heard of, yield little more than half in pig metal, and which

will

will fuffer a wafte of near $\frac{1}{6}$ part to make tolerable good barr iron, and much more, if I am rightly informed, when the iron is intended for more valuable purpofes, fuch as being drawn into wire, &c.

After I had feen his addrefs in his letter to the Society, and his pamphlet; by the affiftance of my friend Mr. Collinfon, I fent him over two or three hints, which I judged might be of fome fervice to him; this produced the favour of a letter from him, of which the following is an exact copy.

To

To Mr. HENRY HORN.

Killingworth, Oct. 4, 1762.

SIR,

I Understand by Mr. Collinson, that you have seen, and greatly approve of, the sample of sand-iron which was sent; that you are desirous to know how it was made, and whether it can be made in large barrs. The little barr you saw, was cut off from a barr of 52 pounds and a half, the first that was made at my son's work, the first that was ever made in America, and probably the first that was ever made in the world, in that manner, and so large a barr. I never heard of any attempt made upon the iron sand, till that of yours 20 years ago, of which Mr. Collinson gave me an account in his letter.

As

As to the manner of making the iron, it is wrought or fmelted in a common bloomary, in the fame manner as other iron ore is fmelted; excepting this dif-ference, this iron fand is fo pure, fo clean wafhed, that there is not a fufficient quantity of cinder or flagg to promote and perform the fmelting, therefore we add either the flagg which iffues from other iron, or elfe add fome bog mine ore, which abounds with cinder; in this way it is as capable of being wrought as rock ore or bog mine.

I was in hopes that if this iron fand could be wrought at all, the particles being fo very fine, it would fmelt very quick; but herein I found myfelf mif-taken, every particle has a will of its own, and muft have its own particular
fmelting,

fmelting, for inftead of its being performed in lefs time, it took more than
common iron ore ; but, upon farther experience, and more acquaintance with this
fand, the workman has fhortened the
operation from five hours down to three:
if by any means it might be reduced to
the fame time with pigg iron, it would
be a moft ufeful improvement. If you
can afford any directions to haften the
operation, I fhould be greatly obliged for
any inftructions.

There is fo much of this fand in America, that I am apt to think, that there is
more iron ore in this form of fand than
in mines.

I have written an effay upon the fubject, which I hope Mr. Collinfon will let
you

you fee, as I hope to fee what you are about to publifh. My fon has a fteel furnace, which was erected feveral years before the act of parliament prohibiting them in the plantations: he has converted fome of the fand-iron into fteel, of which I fend you a fample; as alfo a fample of the iron. As my fon had no inftructions for making fteel, we were forced to hammer out the fkill by various trials as we could; fo conclude that he is ftill imperfect, and wants your help and direction to bring it to perfection, in which art I underftand that you are a perfect mafter, and withal kind enough to offer your affiftance; for which I am very thankful, and look upon it as an additional favour, if you will be pleafed to indulge me with the benefit of your correfpondence, for I live in a corner of the

world

world where fuch information as, I truft, you are able to furnifh, will be highly beneficial. Previous to my attempt of making iron from fand, I propofed my project to thofe who were the moft fkilful in thofe affairs, but met with nothing but what was difcouraging ; yet after all, had a perfuafion of the practicability of the thing to a degree next to enthufiafm, fo that I could not reft till I had made trial. I am glad that the iron has fuch qualities as to meet with your approbation ; I knew that the iron was good, but did not know that it was fo good as your fuperior knowledge has found it. I want to know what fuch iron will fell for in England, whether it will be worth while to fend it. This black fand is a treafure that has long lain hidden from the world, and is

C   what

what may render the colonies more valuable to Great Britain.

I am, Sir,

Your moſt obliged

humble ſervant,

JARED ELIOT.

P. S. The barrs of iron which have hitherto been made of ſand, are from
fifty to fifty groſs, hope in time to have
them reach to ſeventy pounds weight
each ; experience muſt determine that
matter; we can do better than at the
time the eſſay was written. We have
been viſited with a long and ſore
drought, have done nothing for a long
time for want of water.

The ſamples which accompanied this
letter, were two ſmall barrs, weighing
only

only a few ounces, one of the iron made from the fand, the other of fteel made from the fame iron. Thefe barrs I have tried, and found that the barr of fteel worked extreamly well under the hammer, was very pure and clean, and free from flaws. On the contrary the barr of iron turned out much otherwife, for, though it appeared to bear the force of the hammer, as well as the fteel, yet it was not near fo pure, but broke out in flaws and hollows, almoft through the whole of the barr, and which a welding heat would by no means bring into proper union; this however engaged us to try a different method, which was, when the barr was reduced into a proper fize for the purpofe, to double it up three times, one part of the barr upon the other, and to try if it would then bear welding and become more confiftent, and

by

by this means we found the end perfectly well anfwered ; for it bore the
force of the fire and the hammer, and
became in a manner perfectly found.
This fevere trial proved, to a demonftra-
tion, that the iron poffeft all that agreeable toughnefs and ductility, for which
the Spanifh iron is fo defervedly famous,
without partaking of that vile red-fear
quality, for which the latter is very remarkable, and manifeftly tends to prove
the excellency of this fand-iron, when reduced into bar-iron under proper care
and circumfpection.

You will obferve, Sir, from the letter,
that this fand is fo pure, and fo clean
wafhed, that their firft method of reducing the fand to bar-iron proved too
tedious, for want of fome of thofe ad-
ventitious materials, to promote and perform

form the smelting, and which always accompany the common ore, whether it be of the rock or bog kind; which materials, mixing with the matter, made use of by way of flux, and uniting with the ashes of the fuel employed in melting down the ore, is usually run into a thick opake glassy substance, forming, as it were, a covering over the metal, which, by its gravity, naturally sinks to the bottom; this the workmen call cinder. Now the want of this matter rendering the operation too tedious, I find they had recourse either to this cinder brought from other iron works, or to a quantity of the bogmine, which, I doubt not, would abundantly furnish matter for cinder. If they had used only the first, and that properly chosen, it might very probably have been of some service, without doing any material injury to the

C 3   metal;

metal; but if the bog mine is ufed, though the fervice might be apparently more, yet in all likelihood the injury would be infinitely great; and I am inclined to believe that fomething of this kind occafioned the difference obferved between the two barrs above mentioned, viz. that the one might have been reduced by the help of more pure materials, and the other by the affiftance of their bogmine, whofe conftituent parts abound with many impurities, fome of which, by mixing with the metal, may have occafioned the defects above complained of, and which required fo fevere an operation both of the fire and hammer to feparate from it. I am therefore of opinion, that as the profecution of this ufeful difcovery deferves the greateft encouragement, if the Society of arts and manufactures fhould take

it

it under their patronage, the premium they may think proper to propofe fhould rather be given to the perfon who fhall produce the pureft metal, than to him who fhall produce the greateft quantity; for otherwife, I am afraid, we fhall be deprived of what I fhould efteem the moft valuable part of this difcovery; I mean the obtaining a more pure, and better kind of iron, than any we have hitherto been poffeft of, and which I am certain this fand, under proper management, is capable of producing.

I am, Sir,

With the greateft refpect,

Your moft obedient

humble fervant,

Feb. 5, 1763.

Henry Horne.

C 4   OBSER-

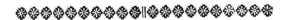

OBSERVATIONS

ON THE

NATURE

OF

IRON AND STEEL, &c.

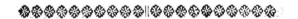

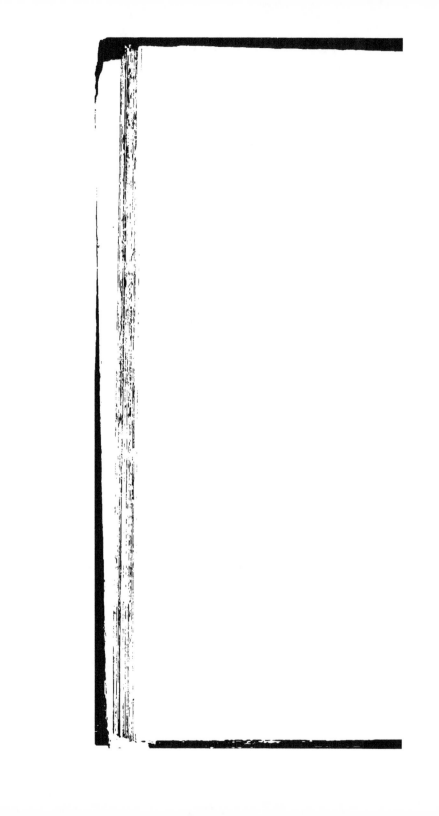

OBSERVATIONS

On the NATURE of

IRON AND STEEL, &c.

SINCE the method of refining steel, first converted in the common way from bar-iron, by remelting it in proper crucibles, and running it into ingots, has been known and practised here in England, where, for aught I can learn to the contrary, the discovery was first made; persons of curiosity have appeared more than commonly desirous of being made a little better acquainted with the nature of this useful procefs. On which account,

C 6 several

several very ingenious and worthy friends have warmly follicited me to profecute a fcheme of this nature. I could wifh, that a perfon better qualified had been pitched upon for fuch an undertaking; however in return for their candid opinion of my poor abilities, I think myfelf under a neceffity of complying with their requeft. And in the profecution of fuch a defign, I fhall review, and make the beft ufe I am able, of a large number of papers, many of which, having been copied as notes upon the trial of a very confiderable number of fucceffive experiments upon the fubject of iron and fteel, have long lain by me.

From this collection I flatter myfelf I fhall be able to felect a number of hints, which (though not arranged perhaps with

with fuch accuracy and precifion as might be expected) may be of fingular ufe in an affair of fo important a nature,

I propofe then in the firft place to make a few obfervations relative to the nature of iron, confidered in its mineral ftate, as it is lodged in, or immediately taken from the bowels of the earth.

I fhall next proceed to fhew the methods which are commonly made ufe of to feparate the metallic atoms from the heterogeneous parts, with which the ore, when firft taken from the mine, always more or lefs abounds.

I fhall after this drop a few felected hints, on the neceffary procefs the workmen are obliged to purfue, in reducing

4   it

it into bar-iron; which will always turn out a better or a worfe fort of metal, according as more or lefs precaution has been ufed in the various ftages of the operation.

We fhall then be qualified to point out, what fort of iron is the moft proper for the purpofe of being converted into good fteel; with the nature of the pro-. cefs by which that change is brought about.

In the laft place, I apprehend, it may not be amifs to give a brief account, both hiftorical and phyfical, of the man-- ner, as well as utility, of reducing the bar-fteel to a more compact and uniform texture, by remelting it in a crucible, and running it into ingots; by which
means,

means, if the operation be well performed, and proper fteel made ufe of,
the metal becomes much better adapted
to the purpofe· of making the fineft edged
inftruments; as razors, lancets, &c. A
very modern method this of procuring
excellent fteel for the above purpofes;
fince no longer ago than the time when
that very accurate writer Mr. Reaumur
publifhed his moft elaborate treatife on
converting bar-iron into fteel, he as well
as others, judged it abfolutely impracticable to melt bar-fteel, without entirely
deftroying its malleability.

But to refume the fubject : in the
profecution of which, my propofed method obliges me, in the firft place, to
take fome notice of iron as a mineral.

Many

Many and various are the accounts of this matter to be met with in our Englifh authors; but moft of thofe accounts, which have fallen under my obfervation, are delivered in terms of darknefs and obfcurity; indeed very fhort hints only, with regard to iron as a mineral, are here and there to be picked up, with little or no connection. Mr. Chambers, in his Dictionary of Arts and Sciences, fays: " Iron confifts of an earth, falt, and " fulphur; but all impure, ill mixed and " digefted, which renders it extreamly " liable to ruft." He then proceeds to give fome very imperfect hints, moft of them trifling, picked up, I imagine, from various unfkilful workmen, who are in general wonderfully fond of noftrums: but thefe, it is my opinion, do not merit any notice.

He,

He next proceeds to lay before his readers an imperfect account of several kinds of iron, as he calls them; but without any real foundation in nature, only as they happen to come from different parts of Europe; from which circumstance he not only presumes to fix their names, but, very unjuftly, to establish their different characters; as fancy, or misinformation, gave him the bias.

This matter I should have passed over in silence, if I had not been in some measure anxious to preserve ingenious and inquisitive persons from being imposed on, for want of better information. Indeed as I proceed, I apprehend I may be obliged to recollect and examine some of Mr. Chambers's hints on this subject, in order to remove some miftakes, which

may

may be judged neceffary to be removed.

From the General Dictionary of Arts
and Sciences, publifhed about twenty
years fince by Mr. Barrow, a few parti-
culars more may be collected. This author obferves, that " true native iron is
" not to be expected in the midft of
" maffes of its ore, but in detached fprigs
" or filaments, in the fiffures of rocks,
" the whole fubftance of which is rich
" in that metal : fuch have been all the
" genuine fpecimens of this rich foffil,
" and fuch their place of formation."
He goes on : " The ores of iron gene-
" rally difcover themfelves to be rich,
" either by their refemblance to wrought
" iron in ftructure and look, or by the
" yellowifh or purplifh tinge they are
" coloured

" coloured with. Thofe which have
" moft of all the appearance of the metal
" they contain, are ufually the richeft."
More hints follow under the fame article, which the reader may confult at his
leifure.

But the moft accurate account I have
met with upon this fubject, taken from
fact and experience, is in a treatife upon
mining, written at the requeft of the late
Duke of Chandois, by one *, who, tho'
the learned differ as to the principles of
his philofophy, was allowed on all hands
to underftand the bufinefs of mining as
well as, if not better than, any man in
England. " Iron," (fays he), " is found
" in thin ftrata of ftone, in nodules

* The late John Hutchinfon, Efq; in the 12th
vol. of his works, p. 187, 183.

" lodged

" lodged fome in, fome between the
" ftrata, in veins, formed in ribs and
" fhoots, in bellies, fome in form of
" ore, fome like clay, and fome by its
" capacity attracted into the moft regu-
" lar and beautiful figures, formed, inde-
" pendent, round from a center, ftriated,
" and compofed of infinitely fmall fpheres,
" divided into fmall cones, fome of them
" having attracted new maffes, and
" formed new centers and arches over
" them in like order; it is feldom found
" native; I have found it very pure, but
" never malleable, or flexible, nor can
" fufion in fire ever make it fo, I think *,
" becaufe

---

* This ingenious writer happens in this remark
to be a little miftaken; for though it is true, that
iron is not to be found malleable in its mineral
ftate; as the vaft quantity of foreign matter, which
frequently amounts to one half of the compound,
keeps

" becaufe it is attracted into maffes; it
" is generally found red, or of a ruft
" colour; in fome places it is found
" black, grey, white, &c. It is generally
" very heavy, and fome of it very hard."
Thus far this ingenious writer.

Poffibly it may be imagined, that
enough has been faid upon the nature of

keeps the metallic atoms fo far afunder as to
render it impoffible to determine, whether, could
they be brought into contact without fufion, they
would be malleable or not; yet, that fufion cannot render it malleable, becaufe it is attracted
into maffes, when run down in the large furnace,
does not prove it abfolutely impoffible to reduce it
by fufion into fuch a form as to infure its malleability. I have myfelf more than once, in fmall
quantities, run it down in fuch a manner, that inftead of being attracted (as this writer obferves)
into maffes, it has affumed a fine grainy appearance; a certain fymptom of malleability : but
then it has always turned out, not malleable iron,
but excellent fteel.

this

this metal, confidered in its mineral ftate; and that we fhould now proceed to give fome account of the means neceffary to free the metallic atoms from the incumbering heterogeneous matters, with which, as taken out of the earth, they are fo very ftubbornly connected. But before I go on to that part of my fubject, I think it highly requifite to remove a difficulty, which moft of our Englifh writers upon iron have left as an obftacle in our way.

I took notice in page 41, that Mr. Chambers, in his Dictionary, hath very arbitrarily affigned names and characters to different forts of iron, according to the different countries where they are produced; this he has done in fuch a manner, (though without any real judgement),

ment), as to give the world a very high opinion of the iron of one country, to the great difparagement of that produced in another.

" There are (fays he) feveral kinds of
" iron, which have properties very dif-
" ferent from one another. As Englifh
" iron, which is coarfe, hard, and brittle,
" fit for fire-bars, and fuch ufes. Swedifh
" iron, which is a fine, tough fort, will
" beft endure the hammer, is fofteft to
" file, and in all refpects the beft to work
" upon. Spanifh iron, which would be as
" good as the Swedifh, were it not fub-
" ject to be red-fear. German iron, com-
" monly called among us Dort Square;
" this is a coarfe fort of iron, and is
" only fit for ordinary ufes." But here

4   comes

comes the cream of the jeft, (if I may be indulged the expreffion,) in the following miftake in fact, and contradiction to what he had before faid. " There is," fays he, " another fort ufed for making wire, " which is the fofteft and tougheft of all: " This is not peculiar to any country; " but is indifferently made, wherever " iron is made, though of the worft fort; " for it is the firft iron that runs from " the mine-ftone, when it is melting, " and is referved purely for this purpofe " of making wire. * "

From fuch miftaken notions of the fuperior value of the iron of one country

---

* Iron wire is, and certainly muft be, drawn from good metal, that is from iron thoroughly cleanfed and well purged; but it makes no dif-ference, as far as I can find, whether it be from the firft, fecond, or laft running.

to that of another, it has arifen, that the Swedifh iron has had the preference given it for making of fteel; and while we have fhewn a fondnefs for particular forts of it, at almoft any price, we have neglected to improve the materials to be found both in our own country, and in our colonies. In my examination before the Houfe of Commons, while the American iron bill was depending, I afferted that this undue preference of Swedifh to other iron, was a mere vulgar error; I repeated it upon oath before the Houfe of Lords; and I now again declare it to be an abfolute fact, that the iron of any country, if properly prepared, is equal to the Swedifh for being drawn into wire, or making fteel; for I have made from our Englifh iron, fteel not at all inferior, if not fuperior, to any that was ever

made

made from the beſt Swediſh; and certain cutlers have chearfully given me for it four times the price at which they could have purchaſed the beſt bliſtered ſteel, made from Swediſh iron: A ſmall quantity of this ſteel I have ſtill by me.

Thus it appears, that the iron of all countries indifferently is fit for the making both of ſteel, and of wire; not for the reaſon Mr. Chambers aſſigns in this latter caſe, namely, becauſe it is the firſt running from the iron-mine; but becauſe it is refined to a higher degree, than is neceſſary for common and ordinary purpoſes; and when once iron is ſufficiently purged to be drawn into wire, or formed into tin-plates, it then becomes extreamly well adapted to be converted into ſteel. The importance of this digreſſion will, I

5   hope,

hope, be judged a fufficient apology for its length.

I am now to fhew the methods commonly made ufe of to feparate the metallic atoms from the foreign matter, with which they are united in their mineral ftate.

I have obferved before, p. 40, that Mr. Chambers in his Dictionary, takes notice that iron in its mineral ftate confifts only of an earth, falt, and fulphur impurely mixed.

The very ingenious Mr. Reaumur, in the beginning of his treatife upon the art of converting bar-iron into fteel, gives a much more accurate account of this matter ; where he informs his readers, that

the

the ores of iron are compofed of ferruginous parts, earthy parts, fulphureous and
faline parts. A more accurate account,
I think, cannot be given of the component parts of iron in its mineral ftate.
" Art," he obferves, " has found out
" the means to feparate the metallic or
" ferruginous parts from the foreign
" ones, with which they are mixed, and
" to reunite and form them into maffes,
" which render them proper for different
" purpofes; to arrive at which," fays he,
" fufion is the firft means to be ufed."
But he fhould have remarked, that previous to fufion it is abfolutely neceffary
to roaft the ore. Dr. Harris, in his Lexicon Technicum, has given under the article of Iron, tranfcribed from the Philofophical Tranfactions, No. 137, or from
the end of a little treatife, entitled,

Mr.

Mr. Ray's Collection of old Englifh Words, the precife method, how this operation is performed at the iron works in the foreft of Dean in Gloucefterfhire. This is done, he obferves, without fufion of the metal, and ferves to confume the droffy part of the ore, and to make it friable. The Doctor here gives a very exact account of the operation ; but does not, I apprehend, completely affign the reafon, which renders it fo abfolutely ne-ceffary ; which is, not only to make the ore friable, but alfo to fet at liberty, and carry off a fufficient quantity of that ftub-born, binding fulphur, which is original-ly inherent in the ore; and thereby render it more difpofed to give up with greater freedom, and confequently in greater abundance, its more valuable contents. Without this operation being made pre-

vious

vious to the fufion, I am ftrongly inclined to believe, from facts I have frequently obferved, that the whole compound would, by the violence of the fire,
run down together into one vitrified mafs,
from which the metallic parts could
fcarcely ever, if at all, be feparated ; at
leaft, not without fo much labour and expence as would render it hardly worth
while to attempt it. The Doctor then
goes on to give a very particular account
of the fmelting furnace, I prefume, taken
from the fame Tranfaction : to which
I refer the reader, to confult it at his
leifure.

I have vifited feveral of thefe fmelting
furnaces in different parts of the kingdom, particularly in Staffordfhire, Yorkfhire, and Suffex. The forms of all I
have

have feen have been pretty much alike, and their methods of working nearly the fame. Notwithftanding which, I have met with very different forts of iron at different places. This, I allow, might in fome meafure be owing to their working upon different forts of ore; but upon the moft fcrupulous obfervation I could make, I cannot be of opinion, for feveral reafons, that this could be always the cafe; for I frequently obferved, almoft at every furnace where I have been, that they worked upon ore fo fimilar in every refpect to that I met with at other furnaces, (and I made the niceft obfervation and the moft particular enquiry I could), that I began ftrongly to fufpect fome latent caufe, not obvious to general notice, muft lie at the bottom of this myfterious affair.

D 4   This

This confideration naturally led me to enquire what fort of flux was made ufe of at different furnaces, and whether the difference of the iron produced might not, in great meafure, be owing to the application of different fluxes. I was pretty foon convinced that my fufpicion was very far from being groundlefs. In Staffordfhire, and fome parts of Yorkfhire, I found that their iron was in fome places extreamly bad, and in others but very indifferent; whereas at feveral of the furnaces in Suffex, I was well affured, their iron turned out much fuperior in quality to what was to be met with in the before mentioned counties. Upon farther enquiry, I became fully fatisfied, that the different materials ufed as a flux, had no fmall fhare in the difference of the iron produced in thefe different parts of the kingdom.

I fhall

I fhall venture to give the reafons of my opinion upon this interefting part of my fubject.

In Staffordfhire, and various parts of Yorkfhire, I found the matter made ufe of by way of flux, was generally unburnt lime-ftone; a fubftance I can by no means think proper for the purpofe. Iron, it is well known, is one of the moft power-ful abforbers of impure acid fulphur in nature; this is fufficiently manifeft from its being made ufe of as a flux for the trying of famples of lead-ore, as well as for the precipitating the martial regulus of antimony. In thefe cafes, it makes a very ftrong, ufeful and purifying flux; as it very eagerly imbibes the impure fulphur, ever to be met with in the lead-ore and antimony in great abundance,

D 5   foon

foon becoming intimately united, and
rifing with it to the furface, where it
forms a very impure fcoria; while at the
fame time, in one cafe, it leaves the lead
pure at the bottom of the crucible; and
in the other, a pure martial regulus of
antimony.

Were we to take it for granted,
that the lime-ftone, ufed as a flux for
reducing and collecting the metallic
atoms with which the iron-ftone abound,
acted in the fame manner as in the cafes
above mentioned, it might perhaps be
fafely made ufe of. But I am well fatisfied, by a great number of experiments
which I have made with the utmoft caution and precifion, that it acts in a manner directly oppofite; for here the earthy
part only of the lime-ftone mixes with
the

the earthy and faline parts of the charcoal, employed in the operation; which
being much lighter than the metalline
parts of the ftone, rifes and fwims upon
the furface of the metal, where it forms
an inert, inoffenfive, glaffy fubftance;
while the noxious, poifonous matter, contained in the lime-ftone, being ftrongly
attracted by the iron, unites and finks
with it to the bottom, and there forms a
rotten, red-fear, bad iron *.

This

---

* In a fmall pamphlet upon fpar, lately publifhed by the ingenious Dr. Hill, he gives an account of the generation of a fluid fulphur in lime-
rocks, in the following manner:

" The primitives of fpar, as we have feen, are,
water, bitumen, chalk, clay, talc and mineral
acid: to thefe the operations of the air, and fire,
give great powers of acting. We thus find heavy
vapours, formed of air, and much water. Thefe
pervading all things, meet the mineral acid, and
uniting with it; if they run clear to the furface,

afford

This I may have occasion to mention again, by way of proof, as I proceed.

I shall now with freedom give my opinion of different substances, applied as fluxes for reducing iron-ore, at other places; and of the propriety with which they are used for that purpose.

In an iron work, at a place called Roberts-bridge, near Winchelsea, and in

afford medicinal springs; but thus united, they may fall upon bitumen. This is no where more frequent than in lime-stone rocks; and often stands in puddles, in their natural hollows. By this mixture, uniting in its course, is formed a real, though a fluid sulphur: for sulphur is nothing else, nor can it be formed by any other means. This sulphur, not yet concreted, passes in its liquid form, through the pores of the lime-stone; dissolving part of its purer chalk as it goes."

If Dr. Hill be right, as I apprehend he is, in the preceding observations, what I have said above, must appear to be the true state of the case.

another

another within a few miles of Tunbridge-
wells, both in Suſſex; they make uſe
of a certain foſſil, to which they give the
name of Greys. Why this foſſil is ſo
called, I muſt leave others to determine.
The materials, of which it is compoſed,
are a congeries of different ſhells of fiſhes,
ſlightly bound together by a ſort of red-
diſh earth, not very unlike ſome kinds of
iron-ore. Large ſtrata of this foſſil are
lodged in the earth, not far diſtant from
theſe two iron works. And it is very
ſafely, and to great advantage, made uſe
of as a kindly abſorbent flux; which being run down with the ore, inſtead of
adminiſtering any bad quality to the
metal, deprives it, in a great meaſure,
of that noxious, arſenical ſulphur, which
too often abounds in its compoſition.
And it may be proper to obſerve, that

the

the iron produced at thefe two different works, is always a fine, genuine, good fort of metal; poffeffed of almoft every good quality, that can be defired.

I fhall mention but one fort of iron more, with regard to fluxes; namely, that which is wrought at the foreft of Dean. This iron, I believe, has been celebrated by almoft every writer upon the fubject, of any confideration. I beg leave juft to recite their feveral opinions; and to tranfcribe an entire paragraph from the ingenious Dr. Harris, in his Lexicon Technicum; a work, in my humble opinion, not excelled, by any of his followers in that way of writing, unlefs by the mere addition of a number of articles, which, at the time when he wrote, had not been fo particularly confidered.

" Iron,

" IRON. In the foreſt of Dean, in
" Glouceſterſhire, the beſt iron-ore is of
" a bluiſh colour, and is called Bruſh-
" ore; but this being melted alone, pro-
" duces a metal very ſhort and brittle:
" to remedy which inconvenience, they
" make uſe of cinder, which is found in
" great quantity where any old works
" have been in that country: for in
" former times, their bellows being moved
" only by hand, their furnaces produced
" a fire much leſs intenſe than thoſe they
" now employ: ſo that formerly they
" melted down only the principal part
" of the ore, rejecting the reſt as uſeleſs.
" This refuſe is the cinder; which being
" mingled with the ore in a due quan-
" tity, gives that excellent temper of
" toughneſs, for which this iron is
" preferred before any brought from
" abroad."

Mr.

Mr. Chambers, before taken notice of, and, I would hope, not unjuſtly cenſured, in his Cyclopædia, expreſſes himſelf thus:

" We have a great number of iron
" works in moſt parts of England; thoſe
" in the foreſt of Dean are in moſt re-
" pute. The ore is found there in great
" abundance, differing much in colour,
" weight and goodneſs.' The beſt, called
" Bruſh-ore, is of a bluiſh colour, very
" ponderous, and full of little ſhining
" ſpecks, like grains of ſilver; this af-
" fords the greateſt quantity of iron,
" but being melted alone, produces a
" metal very ſhort and brittle, and there-
" fore not ſo fit for common uſe. For
" remedying whereof, the workmen make
" uſe of another ſort of material, termed
                                    " cinder,

" cinder, which is nothing but the re-
" fufe of the ore, after the metal has
" been extracted; and which being
" mingled with the other, &c. caufes it
" to be preferred to any brought from
" foreign parts."

This cinder may be confidered in a
twofold capacity; for, as Dr. Harris obferves, the Danes making ufe only of
hand-bellows, which producing, as he remarks, a much lefs intenfe fire, than is
raifed by the bellows now made ufe of;
a confiderable quantity of the metal muft
be left in the cinder, which being again
run down with frefh ore, muft of courfe
be given up; while the other part of the
cinder, may probably yield a very falutary and ufeful flux; for we hear of no
other flux being there made ufe of.

Barrow,

Barrow, in his Univerſal Dictionary, takes but very little notice of this excellent Engliſh iron, comparing it only with ſome iron-ore, found in Hartz-foreſt, in Germany ; which he ſays, is the richeſt iron-ore he knows of, except ſome of the Hæmatites ; but adds, that we have ſome very like it in the foreſt of Dean, which is at preſent worked to great advantage.

The very ingenious and inquiſitive Dr. Shaw, in his notes upon Boerhaave's Chemiſtry, p. 95, ſeems to have copied from Dr. Harris, or rather, perhaps, from the Philoſophical Tranſactions, No. 137, from whence, as before obſerved, Dr. Harris took his hints : and he alſo allows, that the foreſt of Dean iron is preferable to any other.

I have

I have dwelt the longer upon this article of fluxes, as I think it a matter of
the laſt importance; ſince this being well
underſtood, I am fully of opinion, that
we have not the leaſt occaſion to be ſollici-
tous, with regard to any iron imported
from abroad, unleſs from our own colonies; as from thence, or from our own
ore here at home, we may be furniſhed
with any ſort of iron we can poſſibly
want.

It fully appears from the almoſt univerſal ſuffrage of our Engliſh writers, that
from the foreſt of Dean we may be ſup-
plied with iron, ſome ſay as good, others
better than any that comes from abroad.

But poſſibly it may be objected,—
" Taking this for granted, what light
have

have we from thence, relative to the
doctrine of fluxes, (a subject you have
so long dwelt upon), when it does not
appear, that among all that you have
collected concerning the forest of Dean
iron, the word flux is so much as once
mentioned * ?" It is very true, the word
is not mentioned in the printed accounts
I have cited concerning this superexcel-
lent iron. But we are very amply informed, that the brush-ore of the place
is not inferior to the ore of any country
in the world; that this, melted alone,
would turn out very short and brittle;
but being mixed with the old cinder in
a due proportion, it furnishes us with
better bar-iron, than any that comes from
abroad.

* In a paragraph added p. 65, since I wrote this
part, the word is mentioned, and, I apprehend,
with propriety.

In

In every account we meet with of this famous brush-ore in the foreft of Dean, not a fingle hint ever occurs, of the ufe of any other flux than the cinder; and I will venture to affirm, as I know it, from my own experience, to be true, that let a fufficient quantity of this cinder be tranfported to the iron-works in any other part of the kingdom, and made ufe of inftead of the lime-ftone; the iron produced will be nearly, if not equally, as good as that of the foreft of Dean.

If the doctrine of fluxes be not implied in this narrative, I know not where to find it; and if our iron-mafters, as they are called, are not capable of drawing proper inferences from fo plain an account, I am very certain it muft be their fault, not mine.

1 fhould

I fhould now, in courfe, give a few
hints relative to the methods employed
at the forges *, for reducing the fow, or
pig-metal, there melted down, into bar-
iron; but I muft firft mention one interefting particular, namely, the abfolute
neceffity there is, in order to make good
bar-iron, that the flux ufed in the furnace,
be of fuch a nature and confiftence, as to
render it apt and proper to take up as
much as poffible of the common earth,
which greatly abounds in the mine-ftone,
when firft committed to the furnace. If
this be left to be done at the forge, called
the Finery, it muft either occafion a great

---

* Thefe forges are two, which are denominated
the Finery, and the Chafery. They are defcribed
by Dr. Harris in his Lexicon Technicum, and in
the Philofophical Tranfaction before referred to,
No. 137.

wafte

waſte of metal, or the bar-iron will turn out very bad and rotten.

Having premiſed this, I ſhall endeavour to give ſome account of the methods uſed at the forge, called the Finery.

This forge is very properly ſo named, becauſe here the ſow, or pig-metal, is to be freed as much as poſſible from thoſe extraneous matters, which in part conſtitute the ore when committed to the ſmelting furnace; and alſo from an undue proportion of ſuch matter as it may acquire in its paſſage through the ſmelting furnace, either from the flux, or the fuel made uſe of there.

The operations at this forge are well deſcribed in the before quoted Dr. Harris,

under

under the article of Iron, or in the Philofophical Tranfactions, No. 137; to either, or both of which I again refer the reader for his information; confining myfelf merely to point out the confequence of fuch operations, they having a tendency to furnifh us with a better or worfe fort of iron, as they are differently managed.

As this forge then, called the Finery, furnifhes us with very different kinds of iron; owing either to the different forts of ore made ufe of, to the different manner of fluxing the ore, or to the difference in the care and caution of the workmen at the Finery; it may not be amifs to take notice of the different forts of bar-iron, to be met with in the common markets for this commodity, and

the

the feveral denominations under which
the workmen have ranged them.

In general then, thefe different forts
of bar-iron bear the following different
names, as defcriptive of their different
characters, viz. Red-fear, Cold-fear, and
Tough.

Red-fear is of fuch a quality, as to
yield, in a certain degree, to the hammer
when it is cold; but is apt to fly to
pieces under its impreffions at a low-red
heat, and becomes brittle, when between
hot and cold.

Cold-fear is of fuch a nature, as to be
very brittle when it is cold; but it eafily
bears the ftrokes of the hammer when it
is hot, almoft at any degree of heat,

E   *Tough*

Tough is of fuch a nature, as to be very flexible when cold, and capable of fuſtaining pretty harſh treatment from the hammer, either hot or cold.

But among theſe different kinds of bar-iron, are to be found different ſpecies of each ſort: ſome partaking more or leſs of the red-ſear quality, ſome more or leſs of the cold-ſear, and ſome more or leſs of the tough than others.

As the difference of theſe kinds of bar-iron muſt ariſe from different cauſes, it may not, I apprehend, be amiſs to ſpend ſome little time upon an enquiry into theſe cauſes; in order to which, it may be proper to examine what different ſorts of matter enter into the compoſition of what we call iron-ore, or mine-ſtone.

Mr.

Mr. Reaumur, as before hinted, has laid a proper foundation for a full and fatisfactory anfwer to this enquiry, when he informs us, that iron-ore is compounded of two forts of earth, a metallic, and a common one, ftrongly united by falt and fulphur. And I am humbly of opinion, that the falt gives this metal its permanency, while the fulphur occafions its very ftubborn cohefion. It has been before obferved, p. 52,—54, that the fulphur coheres to, and binds the different parts of the compofition together in fo obftinate a manner, that if a confiderable part of it were not diflodged and thrown off by a previous roafting, it would be extreamly difficult, if at all poffible, to procure a proper feparation.

Thus much being premifed, I hope, I fhall now be able to give a tolerable

E 2   account

account of the different kinds of bar-
iron.

The four different forts of matter
abovementioned entering into, and making a part of, the compofition of all iron-
ores, and ftill continuing their connexion,
in different proportions, not only when
they are run into fow, or pig-metal, but
even after they are wrought into bars; it
muft undoubtedly be owing to a more or-
derly proportion of thefe feveral materials,
when the bar-iron proves tough and good;
and to an undue and irregular excefs of
one, or the other of them, when the
metal turns out bad, whether it be of too
red-fear, or too cold-fear a quality: That
this is really the cafe, will admit in fome
meafure even of ocular proof. For inftance: If the common earth abounds in

too

too great a proportion, (which by the way is not easily separable in the usual methods of working), I say, if this exceeds its due proportion, it will infallibly produce a red-sear iron, and the pig-iron of this sort is easily known by its complexion, as it ever exhibits to the eye a very dark grey colour, sometimes approaching almost to a black. The reason why this sort of pig-iron should produce a red-sear iron, when wrought into bars, is extreamly obvious; as well as why it should discover some degree both of softness and toughness, when it is cold; for the common earth being too plentifully mixed with the other ingredients, and being in its own nature softer than the metallic atoms, renders the metal thus compounded, more liable to yield either to the stroke of the hammer, or the teeth

E 3   of

of the file, while it remains cold: But when the more active parts of the composition are put into motion by the force of the fire, the earthy particles, being more subject to dilate and expand themselves, than the more compact metallic atoms; the latter are easily driven to a greater distance from one another, by the expansion of the former; and in this state, I mean while it continues hot, almost the least impression of the hammer will make the parts separate and fly asunder; and thus it comes very properly under the denomination of red-sear iron, whether it be in pig, or in bar. On the other hand, supposing the common earthy particles to be carefully separated, but still an undue quantity of the saline and sulphureous to be left behind; these likewise may keep the metallic atoms too

much.

much afunder, though not at fo great a
diftance from each other, as when they
are too much clogged with common
earth; the confequence in this cafe will
not be the fame as in the former; but on
the contrary, the iron will now be very
brittle when cold; but when heated, and
that to almoft any degree, will fuftain the
moft violent efforts of the hammer. The
appearance put on by the metal in this
cafe, whether in pig, or in bar, is that
of large brilliant and fhining maffes, not
altogether unlike thofe difcoverable in
regulus of antimony when broken. And
here likewife the enquiry is not attended
with any great difficulty, why the bar-
iron arifing from this fort of metal fhould
be cold-fear, as it is called; that is, why
the bars fhould be very brittle when
cold, as well as why they fhould be ca-

E 4   pable

pable of bearing a pretty high degree of heat, and, in that state, of suffering without injury so much violence from the hammer. For as the saline and sulphureous particles, being mixed in too large a proportion among the metallic atoms, naturally, and indeed unavoidably, throw the whole composition into pretty large shining masses, which comparatively suffer those atoms to touch each other but sparingly, and in a few points only; the metal, when cold, must of necessity be very fragile and brittle; but on the other hand, upon a proper application of the fire, as these saline and sulphureous particles are easily reduced to a state of fusion, and as they may be considered as a sort of flux to the metallic atoms, these atoms in this state are brought to be soft and yielding, and easily submit to the

im-

impreffions of the hammer, without fuf-
fering any material injury; and this fort
of iron, if worked with care, is of great
ufe for many valuable purpofes. If the
falt and fulphur be ftill farther difcharged,
but yet fo as that the metal remains cold-
fear in a lower degree, it will begin to
difcover a whitifh, grainy texture, fomewhat refembling the grain of fteel when
broken, after its pores have been clofed
by the hammer; and in this ftate it is
very properly called by the workmen,
cold-fear tough. This grainy appearance
is evidently owing to the metallic atoms
being brought near together, as the ftill
abounding quantity of the other extraneous matter is driven off by the fire,
and preffed out by the force of the hammer. This fort of iron is juftly preferred
by the workmen to the former, as it is

better

better adapted to many more purpofes, and
thofe too of greater ufe. Thus, by ftill
going on to difcharge yet more of the
falt and fulphur, the appearance of the
iron to the eye goes on ftill to vary its
texture; for in proportion as this difcharge is made, the grains are brought
ftill into a clofer contact, and again begin to form themfelves into larger coali-
tions; but of a quite different nature
from thofe which appeared in its cold-
fear ftate; for they now begin to difpofe
themfelves into longifh fibres, with perhaps here and there grains ftill inter-
fperfed; till at length, by ftill carrying
on the operation, the metal is entirely
formed into a fibrous texture; and thefe
fibres become ftill larger and longer, as
the other principles are more and more
difcharged: and in this ftate the iron
becomes duly qualified for all the more

valuable

valuable purpofes, efpecially for the moſt
valuable of all, that of being converted
into the moſt excellent ſteel *. Here it
might not be improper to offer a caution
againſt going too far in this procefs of
refining the iron (though I believe our
iron-maſters, as they are called, are in
very little danger of this, as it would be
attended with a lofs of metal, and confequently with a diminution of their profit) fince by carrying this operation too
far, the iron may again be reduced,
though upon a quite different principle,
to fuch a ſtate as will render it extreamly
brittle, if not quite rotten and altogether.

* If any of my readers are defirous to fee a fuller
exemplification of thefe different appearances, in
the texture of the bars of iron, under the different
ſtages of purification, I would recommend to them
Mr. Reaumur's fifth Memoire, together with the
plate annexed, No. 6.

E 6.   ufclefs,

ufelefs, either hot or cold ; for, a certain
proportion of fulphur being, as before
obferved, abfolutely neceffary to maintain the metallic atoms in a ftate of
union and cohefion, hence, if this vinculum or binding principle be carried off;
the iron muft again lofe its toughnefs
and malleability, and become liable to
fall to pieces under a very flight im-
preffion.

In order to prove, that this would
really be the cafe, I fhall give a fhort re-
cital of an experiment, which I had the
honour to exhibit fome years fince, before the late Martin Foulks, Efq; the then
worthy Prefident, and feveral other re-
fpectable members of the Royal Society.
I ordered a round ball of iron, weighing
about four or five pounds, to be fixed

4   for

for convenience at the end of a long bar of the fame metal. The ball was put into a large fire at one forge, (for there is need of two to make the experiment;) it was there heated to fo great a degree, that it was almoft ready to melt, and indeed till the fulphur, (or cinder as the workmen choofe to call it), was abfolutely in a ftate of fufion. Then being removed to another forge, where there was no fire, and there being dexteroufly applied by one man to the nofe of a large pair of bellows, and another man being placed to blow the bellows, and force the condenfed air with all his might into the pores of the heated ball; in a very few feconds the heat of the ball was increafed to fuch a degree of intenfenefs, as to make the iron drop like melted wax; but fo deprived of its fulphur, which was

thus

thus by the violence of the blaft fublimed and carried off, that the melted metal left behind in a veffel placed underneath to receive it, was become a perfect calx, or crocus of iron. In this manner I have fometimes run off from the ball, four or five ounces of the metal thus reduced to a crocus; in which ftate, if veffels could be procured that would hold, no doubt it would vitrify in a very violent fire, and evince that a very fixed falt ftill remained as part of the compofition, and that the other part was a pure metallic earth; for I am well affured, that by introducing the other principle of fulphur from any proper oleaginous matter, it may again be brought back to the ftate of malleable iron, or fteel, at the will of the operator; and in all probability the refult would be, that the metal thus formed, would turn

out

out the beſt iron or ſteel, that could be procured; as, by this means, it muſt become totally freed from any mixture or remains of the common earth, the great bane of both iron and ſteel.

As a juſt inference from this experiment and its conſequences, I cannot leave this part of my ſubjeƈt, without afreſh inculcating the abſolute neceſſity, in order to make good bar-iron, that the utmoſt care ſhould be taken to extraƈt the particles of common earth, which all iron-ores are ſo exceſſively fraught with; and this ſhould be effeƈted as much as poſſible at the ſmelting furnace, by the application of a proper conſiſtent flux: for if it is not done there, it muſt be done at the finery, where I am certain it cannot be done without a very conſiderable expence of the pure metal.

In

In order to confirm the juſtneſs of this
obſervation, I ſhall tranſcribe a ſhort paragraph from the ingenious Mr. Reaumur,
p. 391. upon the art of ſoftening caſt-
iron, which is as follows :

*Les fontes blanches font plus pures que les
fontes grifes, elles contiennent plus de fer ;
nous l'avons déjà vû, & nous en donnerons
encore une preuve, qui eſt que dans les forges,
on retire plus de fer forgé d'un certain poids
de fonte blanche, que du même poids de fonte
grife. Il y a plus de matiéres étrangéres dans
les fontes grifes, & furtout ; probablement
plus de matiere terreufe, plus de matiere vi-
trifiée de ce qu'on appelle, dans les fourneaux
à mine de fer, du Laitier.* " Pig-iron of
a white colour is more pure than that
of a grey ; it contains more iron ; we have
ſeen this already, and we ſhall give yet
another

another proof of it, which is, that at the forge, they extract more forged iron from a certain weight of white pig, than from the fame weight of grey. There is a greater quantity of heterogeneous matter in the grey pig, and especially, in all probability, more of the earthy, and more of the vitrified matter, of that which they call at the furnaces for iron-ore, Laitier."

As the affair of managing the metal at the forges, is the principal part worth notice, there is room to fay but little as to the manner of their working there; only it may be proper juft to take notice in general, that to the finery, which is the forge of which we have been treating, they bring, as Dr. Harris obferves, their fows and pigs, in order to refine them;
which

which they endeavour to effect in the following manner :

" Into the finery they firſt put the pigs of iron, placing three or four of them together behind the fire, with a little of one end thruſt into it ; where ſoftening by degrees, they ſtir and work them with long bars of iron, and expoſe at different times different parts to the blaſt of the bellows, in order to refine it as equally as poſſible ; till the metal runs together into a round maſs or lump, which they call an Half-Bloom. This they take out, and give it a few ſtrokes with their ſledges ; they then carry it to a great weighty hammer, raiſed by the motion of a water-wheel ; where applying it dexterouſly to the blows, they preſently beat it out into a thick ſhort ſquare.

This

This they put into the finery again; and and heating it red-hot, they work it out under the fame hammer, till it comes to be in the fhape of a bar in the middle, but with two fquare knobs on the ends. This they call an Ancony. Which finifhes the bufinefs at this forge.

" Laft of all it is carried to the other forge called the Chafery, where they adminifter other heats and more workings under the hammer, till they have brought their iron into bars of feveral fhapes and fizes."

Having thus far difcuffed and fettled every thing which feemed to be neceffary upon the article of iron, and clearly fhewn what fort of bar-iron is beft for the purpofe of being converted into good fteel;

my

my method now requires, that I ſhould offer ſome thoughts upon the nature of ſteel.

And here I ſhall endeavour to diſcover its true characteriſticks, ſhew in what it differs from, and in what it agrees, at leaſt with ſome common bar-iron.

Mr. Chambers's account of iron I have already, I hope, not without reaſon exploded: but his account of the nature of ſteel, and the manner of its being prepared, or converted, as it is uſually ſtiled, from bar iron, deſerves, I think, for its obſcurity, a more ſevere animadverſion; unleſs we imagine he had been purpoſely obſcure; judging the ſubject to be of ſuch a nature as it would be criminal to divulge. The ingenious Dr. Harris, in his Lexicon.

Lexicon Technicum, has indeed been more explicit; and what he there offers upon the article of steel, is not only true, but practicable; so far as he enters into the subject. Besides these two, I cannot recollect, that I have met with any English writer, who has offered any thing upon this matter worthy of notice. But it may possibly be expected I should pay some regard to a very celebrated French writer, a late worthy and ornamental member of the Royal Academy of Sciences at Paris, to whose memory I should be unjust, were I not to acknowledge myself greatly indebted to his elaborate performance upon the subject I have ventured to treat of in this imperfect essay: while at the same time I cannot help expressing my concern, that I am under a necessity of differing from him in

that

that part of it, which I am juſt entering upon. But my diſſent even from ſo great a philoſopher will be excuſed, if I am able to give ſatisfactory reaſons for it, founded upon fact and experience. To begin then with iron, in the firſt ſtate in which it may not improperly be entitled to the denomination of ſteel; viz. when it is firſt reduced from its mineral ſtate into what we call pig-metal.

Mr. Reaumur, in the beginning of his 7th Memoire, very juſtly complains, that in the language of common writers upon the ſubject, there is no ſuch thing to be met with as any juſt idea of the nature of ſteel, and wherein it eſſentially differs from iron; that in general the definitions they have recourſe to, are iron more pure, iron more perfect, iron more re-

4   fined.

fined. He names the great Rohault, and adds, that he could mention an hundred others, whose accounts are not more decisive and accurate; upon which he very pertinently remarks; that with regard to the last mentioned definition, that it is iron more refined, it is indeed very faulty; nor will it at all hold good, if we compare it with the idea we have of refining gold, or silver, by which we intend the removal of impure metals, or any other heterogeneous matter which may happen to be incorporated with the gold, or silver. He goes on to make several other very ingenious remarks, well worth our attention; but which we have no occasion to adduce, in order to prove that iron thoroughly purged and refined is by no means entitled to the character of steel; since we have before

us

us fo flagrant an inftance to the contrary, as that pig-metal juft reduced from
the ore, which is the moft unrefined and
imperfect ftate it can be in, is notwithftanding real fteel; whereas bar-iron, refined to the higheft degree for common
ufe, is in the greateft degree remote from
that character, and the more or lefs fo, as
it is more or lefs refined.

But notwithftanding Mr. Reaumur
and myfelf feem perfectly agreed, that
iron-ore reduced to pig-metal is really
fteel, though in a ftate of great imper-
fection; yet the queftion with me is,
how it comes to be fteel?

Mr. Reaumur in his ninth Memoire,
p. 239. in order to give us his idea of
the matter, has recourfe to what he had
advanced

advanced in his firft; That iron in its mineral ftate, is a compofition made up of
earthy particles, ferrugineous particles,
and particles of fulphur, and falt. He
proceeds to inform his readers, that falt
and fulphur abound in all metallic mines;
that the fulphur muft be fublimed and
carried off to a certain degree, before the
metalline parts can be properly feparated.
This, he fays, is the cafe with iron ores,
as well as with the ores of other metals;
which would be liable to great wafte of
metal, if the workmen were not to begin
with roafting the ore, or burning away
by a gentle fire part of the fulphur.

All this is readily granted: but ftill, I
apprehend, it does not quite come up
to the point. There is no doubt that the
ores of all metals in their mineral ftate

F   abound

abound in fulphur; and require this crude fulphur to be carried off, in order to reduce their refpective metals to fuch a ftate of purity and perfection, as will render them fit for their feveral ufes. With regard to different metals, different methods are purfued to obtain this effect. But copper and iron appear to be the two moft difficult metals to be brought to this ftate of neceffary perfection. The former, frequently, requires feveral very elaborate operations for this purpofe; though I have more than once reduced it by one very fimple manner of treatment. After the firft reduction in the common manner of working, it becomes what I think they call black copper; and then it paffes through another operation to render it fine copper, fit for ufe. But my concern is not with copper, but with iron and fteel.

Mr.

Mr. Reaumur is of opinion, and en-
deavours to maintain it with great inge-
nuity, that as the iron-ore contains a very
large proportion of fulphureous and faline
matter in its original compofition, it is
owing only to a partial removal of this
original fulphur, that, in the fucceffive
ftages through which it paffes, it affumes
different qualities, and becomes entitled
to different characters.

Here I muft beg leave to differ from
him : For in my opinion, it is not altogether (if at all) owing to the remains of the
original fulphur exiftent in the ore, that
the metal affumes different qualities in
the fucceffive operations through which it
paffes, but to the introduction of a more
kind and genuine fulphur, difpenfed by
the fuel made ufe of in the operation,

F 2   (I mean

(I mean if the fuel be charcoal) and forced among the metallic atoms by the energy of a violent fire; which either ferrits and drives out the original crude fulphur, and immediately fills its place; or by its falutary virtue, fo far corrects and alters its nature, as to render it innocent and inoffenfive. At the fame time, I am perfuaded, the influence of the charcoal, in the firft operation of running down the iron at the furnace, as truly converts the iron into fteel, as the bar-iron is afterwards converted into fteel, by being enveloped in a bed of materials proper for the purpofe, and lodged together in a furnace as well adapted to carry on and finifh the operation. This perhaps may be made more fully to appear, when we come to treat of that manner of converfion. But when the ofe is

firft

firſt run down at the furnace, the operation being promoted there in ſo violent
a manner, by the ſtrong blaſt of ſuch
enormous large bellows, the ore and the
fuel are ſoon torn to pieces with ſo much
impetuoſity, as to be inſtantly reduced,
both the one and the other, into a ſtate
of fuſion ; when, the former ever eager to
imbibe any freſh ſulphur thrown in its
way, and the latter as eager to perform
its office, one would imagine the ferment
and ſtruggle ſhould be ſufficiently powerful, for the vigorous efforts of the freſh
ſulphur to diſlodge the former foul inha-
bitant, and take poſſeſſion of its place.
And this poſſibly might be more effec-
tually done, if there was no lime-ſtone
made uſe of to promote the fuſion.

Taking this for a true ſtate of the
matter, it muſt neceſſarily follow, that

the

the fteel, thus firft produced, muft be fteel converted to a very high degree, and confequently very hard and fragile; which is well known to be the cafe.

But in order to fhew that in the whole of this I have given a juft account, I muft bring the matter to the teft of experience.

In the numberlefs trials which I have made in miniature, of reducing iron-ore to pig-metal, I have generally been obliged, in order to preferve my crucibles from being torn to pieces, by the voracious quality of the fulphur exifting more or lefs in all the varieties of mine-ftone upon which I have made my experiments, to ufe a certain portion of charcoal duft, the quantity of which I have been ever forced

forced to vary according to the nature
and quality of the fulphur, which I met
with in the different mine-ftone. For
this reafon I have frequently been obliged
to make the fame experiment two or three,
and fometimes four times over; but have
always found, the larger quantity of duft
I made ufe of, the refult of the reduction
was ever a more perfect metal, more
particularly in two interefting experiments.

The firft was that of the American
black fand, an account of which was a
few years fince laid before the Royal
Society, in a letter to my late worthy
and ingenious friend Mr. John Elli-
cott, and by them ordered to be
printed in the Tranfactions. The fulphur
with which this fand was exceedingly

!fraught,

fraught, was of fo fixed, and at the fame time of fo corrofive a nature, that in one inftance upon ufing a pretty powerful flux, the metal was all fublimed and carried up the chimney. In another, where the flux was more moderate, the fulphur carried off the metal another way, by gnawing the fides of the crucible through. But being certain that the fand contained a confiderable quantity of metal, in order to prevent this laft inconvenience, I charged the crucible with fuch a quantity of the duft, that it was difficult, even by the help of the flux, to collect the fcattered atoms of the metal. However, by a little patience and perfeverance, I at laft happily effected it, and was both pleafed and furprifed to find, out of about four ounces of the ore, two ounces of the metal, (though I apprehend not

all

all collected) at the bottom of the crucible; but fo changed, that inftead of
being fine pig-metal, which I expected,
it turned out to be tolerably fine malleable fteel.

But I fhall not enlarge upon this, as I
have reprinted that letter, and prefixed it
to the prefent effay. Nor fhall I here
mention another experiment as much in
point, as this juft now recited; fince I
fhall be under a neceffity of relating it
hereafter.

Now if there is reafon to believe, that
the firft running down of the ore at the
furnace, is really a converfion of the ferrugineous atoms into a very fragile immalleable fteel, I think, it will naturally
follow, that in carrying on the farther

F 5   opera-

operations of refining the metal at the. forge called the Finery, where the fame fort of fuel is continued, and the blaft of a more gentle nature; it will follow, I fay, that the change muft by gentle degrees produce fuch falutary effects, that at a certain period, could the blaft be equally applied to every atom of the metal, as is the cafe in fufion, the refult would be, that the operator would be in poffeffion of a quantity of fteel of a uniform texture, but greatly inferior to fteel converted from good bar-iron; for obvious reafons, which will come in courfe to be taken notice of by and by.

Mr. Reaumur in the above as well as in feveral others of his Memoirs, drops very inftructive hints with regard to the fteel made in Germany, as well as in

fome

fome parts of France, from pig-metal not
reduced to bar-iron, and then converted
into fteel; though at the fame time he
informs his readers, that a more perfect
account of that matter is referved for
another work.

It is to be noted, that this author, in
his firft Memoir, propofes to his readers
three methods of making fteel; the two
firft are the methods ufed in Germany,
and fome parts of France, of making
fteel directly from pig-metal, without its
being firft reduced into bars; his third
and laft method, is that of converting
bar-iron into fteel: and a very odd med-
ley of materials he recommends as proper
to be made ufe of for that purpofe; fuch
as foot, wood-afhes, powdered charcoal,
and fea-falt; and thefe he directs to be

F 6   mixed

mixed up in different proportions, according to the nature of the different forts of iron to be wrought upon. As he profeſſes to found his enquiries upon the practice of caſe-hardening, I am inclined to apprehend that ſome famous practitioner in that way furniſhed him with this notable recipe. The materials may, for any thing I know to the contrary, anſwer very well for the purpoſe of caſe-hardening; but I am not a little ſurpriſed, that ſo great a philoſopher, ſhould ſuffer himſelf to be ſo far impoſed on, as to recommend ſuch a jumble of materials for the purpoſe of converting bar-iron into ſteel: eſpecially as in the courſe of his experiments, he had met with ſeveral ſingle things that would ſo well anſwer the ſame purpoſe, and even mentions the very identical matter generally (if not always) made uſe of.

But

But to bring the matter, as to this point, to a final iffue, I affure my readers, that powdered charcoal alone, or what they generally call charcoal duft, is abundantly fufficient to produce this valuable effect, of converting bar-iron into excellent fteel. This, and this alone, is made ufe of at all the fteel-furnaces, wherever I have been; and I am fully confident that, if this fimple ufeful material were laid afide for Mr. Reaumur's compofition, it would be attended with very difagreeable confequences.

The furnaces made ufe of for this purpofe are of different fizes; fome capable of converting only three or four tonweight, while others are capacious enough to contain from feven to eight or ten tons.

tons. The outfides of thefe furnaces rife
up in the form of a cone, or fugar-loaf,
to the height of a very confiderable number of feet. In the infide, oppofite to
each other, are placed two very long
chefts, made either of ftone, or of bricks
capable of bearing the ftrongeft fire;
which is placed between the two chefts.
The bars of iron, after the bottom is
furnifhed with a neceffary quantity of
charcoal duft, are laid in, *ftratum fuper
ftratum*, with intermediate beds of the
charcoal duft; to fuch a height of the
chefts, as only to admit of a good bed at
top; which is then all covered over, to
prevent the admiffion of the common air;
which, could it procure an entrance, would
greatly injure the operation. The iron
being thus fituated, the fire is lighted;
which is fome time before it can be raifed

to

to a fufficient degree of heat, to produce any confiderable effect. After which it is continued for fo many days as the operator may judge proper; only now and then drawing out what they call a proof bar. This is done by openings, fit for the purpofe, at the ends of the cheft, which are eafily and with expedition ftopped up again, without occafioning any injury to the contents left behind. When the operator apprehends the converfion is fufficiently compleated, the fire is fuffered to go out, and the furnace, with its contents, is left gradually to cool. This may take up feveral days : after which the the furnace is difcharged, by taking out the bars of fteel, and the remainder of the charcoal duft.

The appearance of the bars, as well upon the furface, as in the interior parts,
abundantly

abundantly difcovers the prodigious efficacy of this fimple material, when urged
by a ftrong and fufficiently continued fire.
For the furface exhibits a great number
of tumors, or blifters, which give it the
denomination of Bliftered Steel.

Thefe excrefcences, which we call
Blifters, Mr. Reaumur terms Bulles, or
Boüillons; and apprehends they may be
owing to a fort of boiling, or to a kind
of motion fimilar to that of boiling, made
in the iron; but a little farther on he intimates, that thefe fwellings may be owing
to fome parts of the iron not being fo
well clofed, and rendered compact, while
the bars were under the difcipline of the
hammer at the Chafery. But then it remains a query, Why that fhould be the
cafe? To which, I think, a very ready

anfwer

answer may be given; for as the foul
sulphur, with which the iron frequently
abounds, is not sufficiently purged out
at the Finery, those parts of the bars
where it remains, are with difficulty
brought to unite by welding, as it is
called; and this remaining sulphur being
strongly urged, in the converting furnace,
by the strong fire, joined with the agency
of the more pure sulphur existing in the
materials made use of; must of course occasion a very fierce contest, between the
two combatants; the one endeavouring
to expel the other; which being very
difficult entirely to effect, it is natural to
suppose the consequence must be, that
those parts of the bars which had not
been sufficiently united, may suffer a partial separation, so as to raise these blisters.
What tends to confirm this supposition,

is,

is, that when thefe bars of bliftered fteel happen to come under the hands of a judicious workman; before he attempts to bring them under the hammer, in order to work them down for any requifite purpofe; his firft bufinefs is with a punch, to pierce thefe blifters, (fome of which I have feen near as big as a pigeon's egg) in order to give vent to the contained fulphur, that the iron may be in a ftate, to bear a welding heat, fufficient to bring the parts into a proper union. I have frequently obferved, that when thefe punctures have been made, the air and fulphur have fuddenly rufhed out with a fmart whizzing noife.—Thus much for the change brought about by the converfion upon the furface of the bars.

It now remains to make fome few obfervations, upon the change wrought, by

the

the operation, in the interior parts of the
metal.

Mr. Reaumur is very particular, in
his fixth Memoir, upon this part of
the fubject; where he juftly remarks,
that, as the iron made ufe of, is more
or lefs adapted by its ftructure to be
converted into fteel, the fteel in confequence will exhibit very different phæ-
nomena. It fhould be remembered,
that Mr. Reaumur, and myfelf, are perfectly agreed, what fort of iron is beft
adapted, for being converted into good
fteel; I mean, as to its texture and appearance; namely, that that fort is the
moft proper, which is fo far purged and
refined, as to be formed into long fibres.
During the time of the converfion, thofe
fibres are cut afunder, and after the converfion

verfion fhew themfelves in large fhining
maffes; thefe large maffes, one might expect, would, upon being reduced into
fmaller bars or rods, be again ftretched
out into fmaller fibres. But the change
made in the metal, rendering this impoffible, it may be afked, What is the
circumftance attending this change? A
circumftance, which, though very interefting, appears to have efcaped this
curious and inquifitive writer; but in the
courfe of my bufinefs I have been led to
obferve it. It is this: that upon breaking
a well hammered rod of this fteel; inftead
of breaking off at right angles, with a
faint rotten kind of noife in the rupture,
(which is the cafe attending the common
fort of fteel, converted from ordinary, or
indifferent iron;) this breaks into a long
flaky kind of grain, made up of a longifh

con-

congeries of very fine atoms; and upon
breaking occafions a confiderable concuf-
fion of the air; which the workmen term
a breaking with a twang.

This fort of fteel is much better
adapted to the purpofe of making fine-
edged inftruments, as razors, lancets, &c.
as I fhall have occafion more fully to
fhew, when I come to treat of fteel more
compleatly refined by fufion, under the
influence of a proper flux.

There are two other remarks of Mr.
Reaumur, and others, viz. That the iron,
in paffing under this amazing change of
being converted into fteel, acquires a
confiderable augmentation both as to its
volume and weight.

As

As to the former of thefe, viz. increafe of volume, this ingenious writer
obferves, that what occafions the blifters,
or Boüillons, as he terms them, upon the
furface, muft at the fame time occafion
fomewhat fimilar through the whole body
of the bar; that the effect is fcarcely fenfible, as to the breadth or thicknefs; but
difcovers itfelf as to the length; infomuch that in a fmall bar, only five inches
long, it was increafed one ligne and a
half. As to the increafe of weight, he
makes the amount to be only $\frac{1}{258}$ part
of the whole; in which calculus I apprehend he muft be miftaken; as a gentleman in the north, mafter of a large fteel-
work, has affured me, that he eftimated
his increafe to be one hundred weight
upon feven tons.

I have

I have before allowed an affertion of
Mr. Reaumur's to be juft, viz. That pig-
metal is really fteel, but of a very harfh
fragile nature; though I differed from
him as to the real caufe of its meriting
that character, viz. Whether it is owing
to the raw fulphur originally inherent in
the ore, or to the fulphur of the charcoal
made ufe of in its reduction in the furnace. In order to put it beyond doubt,
that the latter is the cafe, I procured
fome of the moft imperfect fort of Ruffia
bar-iron, termed Brinfky-Iron. This fort
of iron is well known by judicious workmen, to be a compound, of pretty nearly
equal parts, of raw pig-metal, and iron
tolerably well purged; or, according to
Reaumur's opinion, half iron, and half
fteel: I melted a fufficient quantity of
this metal, and run it into an ingot; the

5   con-

confequence was, I had a fmall bar of
low converted fteel, but of an uniform
texture ; which by proper management
however, I had wrought into a dozen of
tolerably ferviceable table-knives. A ftub-
born proof this, that running down in
the fmelting-furnace really converts it
into fteel.

I fhould now have proceeded to perform the promife I made at my firft fetting
out, namely, to fhew the manner and
utility of reducing bar-fteel into a more
compact and uniform texture by fufion ;
were it not for the propriety of firft
taking notice of an extraordinary pamphlet which hath lately appeared, written
by a famous artift in manufacturing fteel
at the weft end of the town; and followed by an advertifement as extraordinary,

dinary, in the Daily Advertiſer, of Wed-
neſday, Jan. 8, 1772. The title of the
pamphlet is, " An Eſſay on the Myſtery
" of Tempering Steel ; wherein the Ef-
" fects of that Operation are fully conſi-
" dered. Said to be extracted from the
" Works of the celebrated Monſ. Reau-
" mur." The advertiſement intimates a
diſcovery being made by this ingenious
artiſt, " of a method of tempering thoſe
" fine-pointed inſtruments called lancets,
" in ſuch a manner as to obviate a gene-
" ral complaint of the liableneſs of ſuch
" exquiſitely fine points breaking in the
" operation."

If ſuch a complaint has been general,
to be ſure, finding out a method to prevent it, muſt be looked upon as a very
uſeful diſcovery. But I never happened

G   to

to be informed before, that it had been general: indeed my own experience muſt bear witneſs to the contrary ; for though I have had great numbers of thoſe curious inſtruments made from my own ſteel, I never heard of one inſtance to favour ſuch an opinion. Indeed happening lately to be in company with a gentleman not long ſince arrived from New-York, he informed me, that in being blooded he had once met with ſuch an accident, the point of the inſtrument having broken in the vein, and been diſcharged by the violent impetus of the blood, iſſuing from the orifice. But being, upon enquiry, informed that the lancet was made by a New-York cutler, my ſurprize was a little abated.

Upon a careful peruſal of the eſſay above mentioned, and looking over the

3

par-

particular Memoir of Mr. Reaumur, from whence the pamphlet appears to be extracted; which before I happened to have taken little notice of; I was concerned to find, what great pains had been taken to make that a myftery, which had before always appeared extreamly obvious, as a matter of fact, and eafily to be accounted for. Mr. Reaumur, I own, has not been fufficiently clear and explicit; having blended together two or three ideas under the fame term, viz. that of tempering of fteel. His tranflator, as he was writing for the information of Englifh artificers, fhould have been careful to have delivered his fentiments in fuch terms, as were familiar to them, and as they could not eafily have miftaken. But this, even at his firft fetting out, he appears to have neglected. He

begins

begins thus : " The diftinguifhing cha-
" racter of fteel, confidered with refpect
" to the offices it ferves, confifts in the
" peculiar property it has of becoming
" hard by means of tempering."

Here the writer confounds two very
expreffive words appropriated to very
different notions; for judicious workmen
generally make ufe of three capital terms,
in order to preferve a proper diftinction of
ideas, viz. Hardening, Tempering, and
Nealing. The firft idea is defined above,
under the term, Tempering; but improperly, for Tempering means reducing the
fteel into a ftate between hard and foft;
which admits of different degrees, according to the different purpofes for which
the fteel is required to be ufed; and is
brought about by adminiftering a differ-

3   ent

ent degree of heat. The laſt, Nealing, is produced by heating the ſteel red-hot, and leaving it, in that ſtate, gradually to cool of itſelf; which reduces, and brings it back, to the condition it was in before it was hardened. By cloſely adhering to theſe terms, we ſhall be able, under every ſtage, to keep our ideas perfect and diſtinct, without running into errors, either on the one hand or the other; or being loſt in myſtery.

The author of the eſſay, in page 4, diſcovers, as he himſelf informs us, the whole of the myſtery in the matter of hardening; which, ſays he, " may be " explained in very few words : A piece " of ſteel is heated, and becoming red, " is ſuddenly plunged in cold water. " This little proceſs," he adds, " is ſuf-

G 3 " ficient

" ficient to have given a confiderable de-
" gree of hardnefs to the piece of fteel,
" which had it been left to remain and
" cool among the coals from which it re-
" ceived the heat, would have been ftill
" in a foft ftate:" that is, it would have
been nealed. As for the myftery, it confifts, I fuppofe, in what he next remarks;
namely, that though the fteel, when, without being plunged in the water, it is left
to cool among the coals, continues in a
foft ftate; yet were we " not pre-advifed
" of the fact, but left to guefs by which
" circumftance the fteel had acquired the
" greater hardnefs, we fhould be tempted
" to pronounce in favour of the latter."
On the contrary, the probability appears
to me to be in favour of the former.
And when I come to affign the caufe of
fteel becoming hard by being quenched

in

in water, I believe it will not appear so mysterious as he imagines. In the mean time, I shall consider the cause which he assigns.

By the " heat," says he, " we give " the steel in tempering" (hardening, he should have said) " we introduce into it " innumerable particles of fire, which se- " parate and detach its parts, and, in " a word, enlarge its dimensions. In " this state," he observes, " it is pre- " cipitated into cold water: the water " very soon puts a stop to the action " of the fiery matter, which had pene- " trated the steel; hence a part of the " augmentation which the fire had oc- " casioned, becomes fixed in the mass." That this is not really a true state of the case, is extremely evident, from the his-

G 4 sing,

fing, and even the boiling of the water, if the body immerfed in it be of any con- fiderable fize; which ebullition continues for fome time, but gradually declines, till at laft it entirely ceafes ; yet not till every atom of the fire is expelled, and forced off through the water. I am very ready to allow that the fteel has an in- creafe as to its bulk, during this opera- tion: but this is owing to quite another caufe than that here affigned ; which will appear, and even be allowed by Mr. Reaumer himfelf, farther on.

He comes in p. 7. to prove, the in- creafed dimenfion of fteel by hardening, from the examination " of a piece of " fteel that is broken after having been " hardened, which," he fays, " will be
" found

" found to be more porous than before:"
and in order to this, he adds a note, extremely curious; namely, " This affer-
" tion muft at firft fight appear extraor-
" dinary," (indeed it muft!) " as thofe
" who have hardened fteel, never think
" that operation well performed, unlefs
" the grain of the fteel appears to be
" much clofer than that in a foft ftate."
It is true, every judicious workman is
really of that opinion; and cánnot well
entertain a different one, whilft he hath
eyes for obfervation.

But what is the criterion by which this
extraordinary pofition is proved ? Why,
by a criterion, in my opinion, as extraordinary as the pofition. For he proceeds thus, imagining no doubt that he
is ftill following Mr. Reaumur: " The

" body

" body of fteel hardened," fays he, " feems
" of a texture much lefs porous than that
" which is not hardened; its grain is,
" neverthelefs, confiderably larger, and
" its appearance of clofenefs is owing
" entirely to the fluid matter which the
" heat had difperfed among its particles,
" and which became fixed in the inter-
" ftices of the grain, by the fudden man-
" ner of cooling it." And if any reader
ftill remain doubtful, he is brought to an
experiment, which is to cure him of his
infidelity. " For he need only quench
" a piece of fteel that is heated much
" more than common, and he will find
" the grain extremely coarfe; for the vio-
" lence of the heat having driven the
" fluid matter from among its interftices,
" the fize thereof will then be very dif-
" cernable."

This

This experiment among workmen is termed burning of the fteel, or rendering it unfit for ufe, without fome farther operation to reftore it to its priftine texture. Many an inftrument have I known thrown away as entirely fpoiled, when this experiment has happened by accident or carelefsnefs.

However, as an experiment, it by no means proves what it is brought for: all it proves is, that if a body of fteel be confiderably heated above what is abfolutely neceffary to give it a proper hardening; the grains, atoms, or fibres, call them by what name you pleafe, are fo far feparated, by the excefs of heat, that plunging them in that ftate in cold water, will not afford a fufficient degree of counteraction, to bring them together

G 6 again,

again, into fo compact a form as to en-
title them to the denomination of fine-
grained hardened fteel. And I think it
extreamly odd, that diftorting a body of
fteel by giving it an over-heat, and thereby a coarfe unconnected appearance, when
hardened, fhould be brought as a proof,
that fteel, hardened in the proper method,
occupies more fpace than before; when
reafons much more conclufive, and more
philofophical, may be brought to prove
the fame fact.

In excufe for fpending fo much time
in confidering this note, and this part of
the effay, I beg leave to make this ufeful
remark : It has been time out of mind
a prevailing opinion, even amongft the
moft experienced workmen, that when
any inftrument, a graver for inftance, is

thus

thus over-heated, it is entirely fpoiled; and accordingly, as before obferved, it is frequently thrown afide as ufelefs; and if the fize of the inftrument is fufficient to admit it, it is cuftomary to carry it to the forge, give it a frefh hammering, to clofe the pores; and then to harden it again, at a more moderate heat. But I can affure my reader, that there is no oc-cafion either to throw away, or to re-hammer, an inftrument thus apparently injured; for if in this ftate it be again committed to the fire, a proper heat for hardening adminiftered, and it be then plunged into the water afrefh, the atoms will be brought together again in the moft cordial manner, and form as fine a texture, as can be defired; and yet the fteel will occupy more fpace than it did before it was hardened.

The

The truth of the cafe is, that if the heat be too low, the fteel will not receive a fufficient degree of hardening by being plunged in the water; if it be over-heated, the parts will be removed to fuch a diftance from each other, as to render the check it receives from the plunging in the water, infufficient to reftore them to a proper contact, fo as to render it fit to form a fine inftrument: but neither in the one cafe, nor the other, is the fteel itfelf really injured, the conftituent parts remaining ftill the fame; fo that if it be heated a third time to a proper degree only, and then replunged, it will receive as fine a grain, as if the firft heat had been adminiftered with all imaginable ac-curacy. This fecret I was acquainted with, many years before I knew any thing of Mr. Reaumur: I have yet, fo far as I

can

can recollect, communicated it only to two ingenious mechanics ; but having the prefent opportunity, I thought it my duty to make it public.

I hope to be excufed if I pafs lightly over the remaining pages of this performance, and leave my readers to an attentive perufal of the effay itfelf, if they think it requifite.

In page the 9th is only a trial made by Perault, retried by the effayift, to prove the enlargement of fteel by tempering, as he calls it ; a thing, which I apprehend, nobody denies.

The next page contains a calculation made by Mr. Reaumur, of the amount of that augmentation which fteel acquires

by

by hardening; namely, a 48th part at least of its original size; which I presume likewise, no one will controvert. The writer's inference, I own, I do not understand, viz. " That what he has before " offered sufficiently proves, that tem- " pered steel is of a texture more rare " than when it is soft." If by more rare, he desires to be understood, that the parts of the former are more separated and detached the one from the other, than they are in the latter, I can by no means agree with him : and if the former experiment of over-heating be again brought as a proof; I cannot help saying, that it is really nothing more than a mere *deceptio visus.*

After a number of experiments made to prove, that the increase of the hard-

nefs of fteel, notwithftanding the augmentation of its fize, is not owing, either
to the fire or water adding any matter to
the fteel, which occafions the increafe,
and unites its parts better together; or
to its driving any matter out of it, which
prevented the parts from being fo well
united as they might otherwife be; all
which experiments appear to me very in-
fignificant, notwithftanding Mr. Reaumur
himfelf feems to have given them a
fanction: after all this, I fay, at the bottom of the 22d page, the writer brings
the affair to a crifis.

He there obferves what, he fays, " is
" well known, that the principal diffe-
" rence between iron and fteel is, that
" the latter is very confiderably more
" impregnated with particles of fulphur
" and

" and falt, than we find the other to be."
Here then we are to find the precife difference between the two; and at the fame
time, the reafon why, and the manner
how, fteel acquires the property of becoming hard. But how comes it to pafs
that we could not at once have been
brought to this criterion, without being
led through fo many obfcure and intricate
windings? Would the myftery, as he af-
fects to call it, have appeared lefs fur-
prifing?

We are next reminded, that both iron
and fteel have an aptnefs to imbibe fulphur, as they acquire heat: This is extremely well known, and is true not only
with refpect to iron and fteel, but likewife every other metal; or copper would
never be converted into brafs by being
in-

in a proper manner mixed with a due
proportion of *lapis caliminaris*; nor would
it become what is called bell-metal by a
proper mixture with tin. But to return,
the premiffes being admitted, what is the
confequence? To determine this, we are
to call in, it feems, the aid of the mi-
crofcope, in order to difcover the component parts of fteel; a fingle grain of
which, we are told, is made up of a collection of other grains, which we are to
term molecules; and thefe appear likewife to be made up of other parts, which
we are allowed to fuppofe are of an elementary nature. And he tells us, p. 24,
that " to carry our ideas fo far as the
" fubject would permit, we might ftretch
" this divifion much further; but it may
" be fufficient for the prefent purpofe to
" let it reft here." And then he informs

us,

us, what ufe he makes of this minute divifion, in order to explain more fully, " how
" fteel becomes hard, when it is cooled
" fuddenly, and why it is foft, when it is
" fuffered to cool by flow degrees." His
words are thefe, which I quote at length,
that I may not, by abridging, mifrepre-
fent them : " We have, fays he, under
" our confideration a fingle grain of fteel,
" the molecules it is compofed of, and
" the elementary parts of thofe molecules.
" Now, in expofing to the fire the piece
" of fteel which contains the grain (at
" prefent the object of our confideration)
" we fhall find, that the fulphur and falts,
" contained in the molecules, will be
" fooner melted than the molecules them-
" felves, and are by the heat driven from
" among the parts in which they were
" contained, and take place amidft its
" vacancies.

" vacancies. Thus the matter, which the
" heat had expelled from within the mo-
" lecules, now fills up the fpaces between
" them : it is pretty evident then, that,
" when a grain of fteel has received a
" certain degree of heat, the vacant fpaces
" of the molecules, of which it is com-
" pofed, are in part filled up by a ful-
" phurous matter, which they did not
" before contain, and which had been
" extracted from the molecules them-
" felves. In this ftate the piece of fteel,
" which contained . the forementioned
" grain, is fuddenly plunged in water,
" and, in that inftant, we fix at once the
" fulphur and falts, which were in a ftate
" of fufion, and thereby depriving them
" of their fluidity, they are no longer in
" a condition to re-enter the cells, from
" which they were driven. And thus,"
fays

fays he, " the fmall interfpaces of the
" molecules are better filled up, and by
" a matter which we may fuppofe almoft
" as hard as we pleafe." But is it not
obvious to remark, that if the interfpaces
between the feveral molecules are thus
filled up by a fulphurous and faline matter, which is derived from within the
molecules themfelves, and which muft
be fuppofed to be, as it were, the cement, which unites the elementary parts
of the molecules together; then in proportion as the exterior parts of the feveral
molecules are more united to one another, and become harder, the interior elementary parts, being deprived of this cement, will become lefs united with each
other, and be more eafily feparated. All
the effect, therefore, which I can perceive
likely to follow from a different pofition

of

of the fulphurous and faline matter, which is fuppofed to be contained in the feveral molecules, will be the diffolution of the old molecules into their elementary parts, and the forming new molecules of other elementary parts, united by that fulpurous and faline matter, or cement, which, before it was driven out of its place by the heat, united the parts of the former molecules. In fhort it appears to me impoffible, to account for the hardening of fteel, merely by the removal of the fulphurous and faline matter from one part of it to another; fince what is thus gained in one part, will be loft in the other. I apprehend, therefore, we fhall be obliged to have recourfe to the introduction of a certain quantity of fulphurous and faline matter, in order to account for this phænomenon: of which I fhall treat more largely hereafter.

The

The writer, p. 29, not very happily
indeed, falls upon cafe-hardening, as the
fitteſt ſubject to exemplify his ideas; adding a remarkable note, to explain what is
meant by cafe-hardening. " This opera-
" tion," ſays he, note, p. 30, " is termed
" by thoſe who perform it, cafe-hardening,
" and with much reaſon, as the thing,
" which is to be hardened, is heated in a
" cafe, uſually made of iron." This happens to be *un faux pas*; and I hope the
gentleman will not take it amiſs, if I endeavour to ſet him right. The term
then is made uſe of to intimate, that by
the operation (which he explains tolerably
well) it is intended to cover the ſubject,
whether it be a bar, or any particular inſtrument made of iron, with a coat, or
cafe of ſteel, thicker, or thinner, at the
pleaſure of the operator, as the operation

is

is continued a longer, or a shorter time: and he might as well, for the reason he gives, have called converting bar-iron into steel, case-hardening; since the bars to be converted, are likewise confined in a case.

A little farther on (p. 32.) he remarks, that " This method" (namely the operation of case-hardening) " used even with " iron, occasions a hardness about its sur- " face, approaching to that of steel," and as he expresses himself afterwards, " nearly equal to that of steel." I must beg leave to inform him, that the hardness thus occasioned, is quite equal to that of steel; and that the surface of the metal is really steel.

In a note in the preceding page he saith, " This process, however, is com-

H   " monly

" monly ufed with iron only, fteel being
" capable of receiving a fufficient degree
" of hardnefs by the methods ordinarily
" practifed for that purpofe." A very odd
remark this ! What, are there two different methods made ufe of, the one to
harden an entire piece of fteel; and another to harden a piece of iron cafed over
with fteel? For my own part, I never
heard of more than one.

" This procefs, however," he tells us,
" is commonly ufed with iron only."
But it has been ufed with fteel alfo ; and
poffibly I was myfelf the firft that fo ufed
it. And I would here inform the effayift,
that as a cafe of fteel, may be formed
upon a rod of iron; fo a cafe of harder
fteel may be fuperinduced upon a rod of
already converted fteel.

When

When making artificial magnets firft became pretty much in practice, I among others was willing to have a ftroke at it, and being as willing to excel, I ufed the method of cafe-hardening the bars; by which I found my bars really did excel. And the late Mr. Canton, who was fo lucky as to hit upon a more expeditious method of communicating the magnetic virtue than had before been practifed, was affifted by me in procuring the beft bars for his purpofe. I gave leave to a very ingenious and worthy man, then in my fervice, (without receiving any benefit myfelf) to employ his leifure hours in forming and hardening bars for Mr. Canton, according to a method which I had directed, and with the nature of which I made that gentleman acquainted, upon his applying to me, previous to the pub-

H 2   lication

lication of his account of the manner of making artificial magnets, in the Philo-fophical Tranfactions. To this method of hardening the bars, the knowledge of which he received from me, Mr. Canton refers, when he *coolly* fays, (I wifh he had expreffed himfelf in more friendly terms,) the fmith that I *employed*, hardened them fo and fo.

If the effayift had followed his author into the next Memoir, he might have met with obfervations worthy his notice ; and perhaps the more fo, as fome of them are flat contradictions to thofe hints, from which he had drawn fome effential con-clufions. Particularly, whereas, p. 40, he fpeaks of " fteel becoming harder by " being tempered hotter," Mr. Reaumur obferves, p. 344, that it has been an ob-fervation

fervation of fome curious workmen, that when fteel had been tempered, or hardened, at too hot a colour, it would not render it more, but rather lefs hard, than when heated to a more moderate degree; and I apprehend this to be the fettled opinion of every one, who merits the name of a good workman.

I hope I fhall be excufed having led my readers fo far out of the way in queft of an imaginary myftery in tempering of fteel : I fhall now lay before them briefly the true ftate of the cafe; that if there be any myftery, we may be able to give it a proper inveftigation.

I allow with Mr. Reaumur, that when the iron-ftone is firft taken from the earth, it brings along with it a very foul

H 3   fulphur;

sulphur; to remove which in some measure, before it enters the smelting-furnace, they are obliged to give it a strong
torrefaction; in which operation not only
a great part of the sulphur is expelled,
but the body of the mineral, (as before
observed) is so far opened, and the stub-
born texture of the compound, occasioned
by the crude sulphur which strongly binds
it together, is so far relaxed, that when it
comes into the furnace, the remainder of
its natural vitious sulphur suffers an easy
expulsion, by the large quantity of charcoal made use of in the operation, assisted
by the strong blast of the bellows; while
at the same time the more kindly sulphur
of the charcoal supplies its place, and
converts the metal into a very hard frangible steel.

In

In the fucceeding operation at the forge called the Finery, if any of its original fulphur yet remain, of which I apprehend there can be only a very inconfiderable quantity, that likewife fuffers a very eafy fublimation ; but it happens at the fame time, that not only the remainder of this crude fulphur, if there be any, but likewife a very confiderable quantity of the more falutary falt and fulphur, which it had recently imbibed from the charcoal, unavoidably makes its efcape, along with it ; becaufe, (notwithftanding the fuel ftill made ufe of be charcoal,) the operation is performed in a more gentle manner, and upon an open hearth.

In the courfe of this operation, the metal through every ftage for a confiderable time ftill retains the character of

H 4   fteel ;

fteel; but of a higher or lower degree,
in proportion to the quantity of fulphur,
that has in this manner been carried off,
till at laft it becomes malleable fteel:
all this Mr. Reaumur allows to be true;
and he farther obferves, that could the
metal be in every part uniformly and
equally applied to the blaft, it might at
a certain period be deemed tolerably good
fteel.   But as this equality is in this manner very difficult, if ever, to be obtained,
it has been judged neceffary to carry on
this operation ftill farther, to reduce the
metal to fine malleable bar-iron, in order
to its being in a proper condition, to be
reconverted into bar-fteel.

But how is this recovery, or reconver-
fion, to be obtained? Why ftill by the
medium and miniftry of charcoal: and
the

the manner in which this is effected, is
shewn in a former part of this essay, p. 109,
&c. where the nature of the furnace, in
which the operation is performed, and
the process itself, are fully described, as
well as the changes, both external and
internal, which are made upon the metal.

And now as to the mystery of tempering, from every observation that can
be made between the different natures of
iron and steel, I am obliged to subscribe
to what Mr. Reaumur himself has advanced upon the subject, viz. That one
differs from the other merely in being
impregnated with a larger proportion of
salt and sulphur. At his first setting out,
in his treatise upon the art of converting
bar, or forged iron into steel, he affirms,
as I have frequently observed, that the

H 5   mines,

mines of iron are compofed of ferrugineous parts, of earthy parts, and of parts of fulphur and falt. It has been already fhewn, that a method hath been difcovered to feparate the metallic parts, or ferrugineous atoms, from the heterogeneous matters with which they are mixed, and to reunite, as Mr. Reaumur obferves, the parts difperfed into a proper mafs, to render the metal fit for its feveral different ufes. He proceeds to obferve, that fufion is the firft mean employed for this purpofe.

Now if from what has been offered, we may venture to take it for granted, that at the firft running down of the mine, by means of the large quantity of charcoal made ufe of in the operation, the iron is converted into a very hard immalleable, and to the higheft degree frangible, fteel: which

which Mr. Reaumur himfelf allows to be
the cafe, and even makes it the firft
term of his gradation, when enumerating
the various degrees of fteel in refpect to
its different hardnefs: and if this difference, as he allows, be owing to one
degree being impregnated with a larger
proportion of falt and fulphur than the
other; from its ftate of pure malleable
iron, with only fo much fulphur left as is
fufficient to form a vinculum, to hold
the parts of the metal in a proper degree
of cohefion, to the higheft term in his
gradation: I fay, allowing this to be true,
I cannot help being of opinion, that every
degreé of the converfion of bar-iron into
fteel, from the loweft term to the higheft,
carries on in the metal a fucceffive ap-
proximation to the nature of a femi-
vitreous body. Pig-metal, as it is called,

H 6   is

is almoſt as hard, and nearly as fuſible as
glaſs. Bar-ſteel highly converted, and
formed into a proper inſtrument, will cut
glaſs almoſt as readily as a diamond. A
bar of high converted ſteel being broken,
and compared with a bar of pure iron,
the former exhibits a very different appearance from the latter; the one is eaſily
brought into fuſion in the crucible; the
other, with the greateſt difficulty; and
ſcarcely at all, if very pure. I have myſelf frequently made the attempt; but
without ſucceſs; as I have ſcarce ever
been able to reduce it to a ſtate of fluidity; inſtead of which, I have been able
only to tear the metal to pieces, by ſuch
a diſunion of its parts, that when I have
attempted to run it into an ingot, it has
run out of the crucible moſtly in a fine
ruddy powder, with here and there a few
ſmall

fmall maffes clinging together very loofly. And to compleat the whole, when it comes to be hardened, by being properly heated, and fuddenly quenched in cold water, it becomes almoft as brittle as glafs itfelf; and by a proper admixture of other matters, affifted by a flight previous calcination, it may with no great difficulty be run into glafs. And here, if any where, I am fully of opinion we muft look for the great myftery (not of tempering, but) of hardning fteel: which may be briefly explained in the following manner:

Steel is iron converted, as it is properly termed, by the introduction of a certain quantity of falt and fulphur; which, being not only mixed and fettled between the interftices, but entering into, and even

making

making a part of the minuteſt atoms of the metal ; and being, at the ſame time, by a very moderate degree of heat eaſily brought into a ſtate of fuſion, ſwells and expands every atom of the metal; and the metal in this ſtate being ſuddenly im‑merged in cold water, every atom, with its contents, is as ſuddenly arreſted in this expanded ſituation, which, at the ſame time that it increaſes and fixes its bulk, renders it nearly as brittle as glaſs.

Having thus far (I hope ſatisfactorily), cleared the way, with regard to the myſtery, as it has been fondly termed, of hardening ſteel ; I ſhall now ſubjoin a few conſidera‑tions, with regard to the myſtery, if it muſt be ſo called, of tempering ſteel.

This among our Engliſh workmen is termed, and I apprehend not improperly,

reducing

reducing or letting down, that is lowering, the nature of the steel, by administering such different degrees of heat, as may be proper to qualify the instrument to which it is applied, for its intended use.

Thus, for instance, with regard to razors, lancets, and such curious instruments, the custom is, either by an open fire, or by a red-hot bar of iron, to apply the instrument to the heat, and hold it there till the proper colour, by which to judge of the heat given to the instrument, appears upon the surface, as perhaps a high gold colour; and then the instrument is again immersed in the water, as suddenly as when it was at first hardened; this is done in order again to arrest the phlogiston in its then state; as otherwise,

7. the

the heat, remaining in the metal, would
go on ſtill farther to reduce the temper of
the inſtrument, till it would be diſqua-
lified for the purpoſe intended. If the
inſtrument be of a groſſer kind, the colour muſt be ſtill farther advanced, and
the temper ſtill farther reduced, till the
inſtrument be judged fit to endure the
more arduous work it is intended to perform.

But as no ſubject, that I know of, requires a more accurate adjuſtment and
preciſion in this particular, than the
ſprings of watches; I ſhall ſingle out
that, as one of the moſt intereſting, to
give it a very cloſe and impartial con-
ſideration.

The main ſpring of a watch is known
to be a very thin plate of ſteel; in this
form

form it is brought into a double ring, bound round with wire, and committed to a proper furnace, in order with great caution to give it a fuitable degree of heat; when that is fufficiently acquired, it is taken out, and dropped into a kettle of oil, or warm mutton fuet; for water would prove too chilling; from hence being taken out, it has acquired a degree of hardnefs, very little inferior to that of glafs. After this it is reduced, or let down, if the fteel be of a proper kind for the purpofe, to a fine violet, or blew colour; in which ftate it becomes excef-fively elaftic, infomuch that to make it to ftand bent, it muft be brought into a very acute curve; nor can it eafily be brought by twifting horizontally to alter its form, without endangering its being rent to pieces. But as after this, it re-

quires

quires to be planifhed by the hammer,
filed and polifhed, it again becomes deprived of its elafticity to a very confiderable degree; but when it has received
its laft degree of fine polifh, it is again
blued upon a brafs plate over a lamp, by
which means its former elafticity is perfectly reftored.

What is here extremely remarkable is,
that had the fpring been wound up, and
placed in its proper inclofure in the
watch, without being again blued; it is
much to be queftioned, whether the watch
would ever have meafured time with any
tolerable degree of exactnefs; yea, fo abfolutely neceffary is the retention of this
blue fkin, if I may fo call it, upon the
furface of the fpring, that if ever, by the
inequality of the fpring, a more than ordinary

dinary friction fhould happen among the turns, fo as to rub off the fkin in any confiderable number of places, which I have frequently known to be the cafe; the elafticity will become fo vehemently difturbed, that the watch will never afford any proper degree of fatisfaction to the wearer, till the old fpring be removed, and a new one placed in its room. The ingenious Dr. Hook, in his Micographia, taking particular notice of this fine blue covering, gives it, very pertinently, as his opinion, that it is owing to the fine fulphur, preffed through the pores by heat, and fixed by the ambient air in a fine vitrified lamina upon the furface.

It would, I think, be a very curious, as well as interefting, query: What is the phyfical

phyſical reaſon of the variation of elaſticity under this variation of circumſtances ?
the elaſticity of the ſpring, upon the firſt
tempering of it, being prodigious; and
in the operation between the tempering,
and its acquiring the laſt fine blue
covering, being very conſiderably dimi-
niſhed; and, by introducing the laſt
covering, being again amply reſtored
and fixed.

Having now ſaid every thing, which I
apprehend neceſſary, relative to the nature of iron; tracing it from its being
firſt taken from the mine, through every
ſtage, till it is reduced to good bar-iron;
and having likewiſe diſcovered what
change is wrought upon it, in its con-
verſion into that ſtate, in which it aſſumes
the denomination and character of ſteel;
and

and marked out the difference between the one and the other; I now proceed to confider, as I propofed, both hiftorically and phyfically, the lately difcovered method, of re-melting bar-fteel in a crucible, and running it into a folid ingot; by which means, when the metal is properly chofen, and the operation duly performed, we are furnifhed with a more excellent kind of fteel, for fome important purpofes, than was probably before known in England.

It is not a great many years fince this difcovery was firft made, by a gentleman (as I have been informed) refiding in the Temple, an acquaintance of the late Lord Macclesfield; whofe name I could never learn; nor could I ever gain the leaft information of the means, by which he be-

came

came poffeffed of fo valuable a fecret.
He however judged it proper not to let
it remain a fecret any longer, than till an
opportunity offered of difcovering it to
fome perfon, who, he imagined, might
be able to render it of fervice, in fome
fhape or other, to himfelf, as well as to
the world. While the gentleman was
thus inclined, there fell in his way, one
who had been employed in flatting of
gold and filver wire for the ufe of the
lace-men; whom he judged to be a proper perfon for his purpofe.

Prior to this period, the workmen at
a very confiderable expence, and no fmall
rifk, had been obliged to fmuggle thofe
implements, or fteel-rollers, by which
the wire is flatted, from Lyons in
France; whereas our melted fteel is
qualified

qualified to form them in a much better manner; but ftill liable to this confiderable objection; that as the fteel is obliged firft to be forged into plates, there is an abfolute neceffity of their being welded in one particular part, which not only injures the fteel, when they are bent round the iron roller, but leaves a difagreeable roughnefs upon that part, where the welding-heat muft of neceffity be adminiftered.

To obviate this difficulty, the ingenious Dr. Lewes has propofed a more advantageous method of forming thefe rollers, viz. By having them caft in one entire piece, with a proper opening in the centre, by which means they may very commodioufly bear the difcipline of the hammer, in order to clofe the pores, that they may become fit for being hardened.

Hap-

Happening lately to fall in the way of my ingenious friend Mr. John Bird; who difcovered fome concern with regard to the difficulty of procuring a couple of fteel collars, to turn upon the cylinders at the centers of the large quadrants, which he was than making for the new Obfervatory at Oxford, without being fubject to wear by the friction; this hint of Dr. Lewes's fo forcibly ftruck me, that I immediately propofed their being formed in this manner; the attempt fucceeded fo well, that I became thoroughly fatisfied, Dr. Lewes's fcheme might eafily have been put in practice, could one difficulty have been fufficiently guarded againft, namely, the liablenefs there might be in the rollers to caft, or fly in the hardening. This difficulty has fince been overcome by Mr. Bird, the ingenious artift juft mentioned. To return:

The

The person, to whom the secret above-mentioned had been communicated, could not rest satisfied with a vigorous pursuit of his own business, the flatting of gold and silver wire, which might in all likelihood have proved very advantageous to him ; but must needs, though no competent judge of the nature either of iron or steel, commence a maker of razors ; imagining, I presume, that nothing more was necessary to form a good instrument of that kind, than its making a fine brilliant appearance. For this purpose, having melted a considerable quantity of steel, without being a judge whether or not, it was fit for the purpose ; he applied to a very honest worthy man, one Mr. Humphrys, a cutler near Covent Garden, who for a suitable premium became his operator.

The

The razors, made from this fort of steel, wearing, whatever was their intrinfic merit, a much finer face than common, procured him a pretty large number of cuftomers at the weft end of the town, where he became a confiderable hawker. This circumftance foon alarmed the cutlers in that part. Upon which old Mr. Savigny, a very ingenious artift in his way, the above named Mr. Humphrys, with feveral others whofe names it would be needlefs to mention, applied to me ; and at their entreaty, having built a furnace, I went to work ; and though at firft fetting out I met with no fmall difficulties, it was not long, before I was enabled to furmount them, and to furnifh my folicitous cuftomers with a commodity, vaftly fuperior to what the perfon, who had rifen up in their way, had fufficient fkill to procure for his own ufe.

I and

I and my new cuftomers went on cordially for fome time, as I had undertaken to ferve them at a very moderate price. But it fo happened, that our razor-maker, finding the large expectations he had formed in this new employment, broken in upon by my cuftomers, who were qualified vaftly to outdo him ; foon fell upon a new fcheme, by which he apprehended, he might both injure his competitor, and procure himfelf great advantages. For this purpofe, he went into the North, to difpofe of his fecret to the beft advantage ; firft to Birmingham ; and not finding fufficient encouragement there, to Sheffield ; and, as I have been informed, offered his fecret to feveral confiderable manufacturers, at fo extravagant a price, that few or none cared to be purchafers. However, he met a ſo th fome keen friends, who wormed the fecret cut of him, fupplied him with a little money, and fent him back to town; and they, being better fkilled in the nature of fteel than he was, foon outdid their mafter. My new cuftomers, now finding they could purchafe melted fteel from Sheffield at eight or ten-pence a pound, difpatched their orders thither, without any regard (which is too common a cafe) to the trouble and expence, which at their own requeft I had been at, to ferve them under their difficulties. What advantage this exchange hath been of to our London artificers, I fhall not pretend to determine; they beft know, or ought to know, whether it hath been of any, or the contrary. But certainly, the difcovery of this affair at Sheffield hath turned out of great fervice to that large and

populous

populous feat of manufacturers; which wears, as I have been well informed, at prefent, a very different afpect from what it did not many years fince, before it was in poffeffion of this new and valuable branch of commerce.

Thus have I given a brief hiftorical account of this recently difcovered art of reducing bar-fteel by fufion, into a more compact and uniform texture.

As to the phyfical nature of the change wrought upon this ufeful metal by the new manner of reduction; I fhall be but fhort upon it; and perhaps not quite fo explicit, as fome perfons, for their own intereft, may wifh me to be.

It has been obferved in the beginning of this effay, that no longer ago, than

I 3   when

when Mr. Reaumur publiſhed his treatiſe
upon converting bar-iron into ſteel, which
method of coming at that valuable metal
he juſtly prefers to every other; I ſay at
that time, this new method of operation was judged to be very difficult; nay,
he pronounces it abſolutely impracticable.
I own, I was then ſo far of his opinion,
that I ſhould ſcarce ever have ventured
upon ſuch an attempt, if the practicability of the operation had not been made
apparent by its having actually been effected by the perſon I before mentioned,
and if I had not likewiſe been ſtrongly
ſolicited to make the experiment.

What might poſſibly lay a foundation
for the opinion of its being impracticable,
might be the accident, before taken notice of, which ſometimes happens at the
con-

converting-furnaces; when by fome im-
perfection in the pots, or chefts, the grofs
air finds a paffage in among the contents;
which is ever fure to demolifh a confiderable quantity of the metal, if running
it down into grofs lumps may properly
be called a demolition.

Some years fince, a very fenfible man
fell in my way, who had many years been
employed at Mr. Crawley's works at Newcaftle; this perfon informed me, that accidents of this nature fell out, not un-
frequently, at their fteel-furnaces in that
place; and that great quantities of this
reduced metal, which he had ever obferved to be as hard and obdurate as pig-
metal itfelf, had been buried in the earth
to prevent a difcovery, leaft the workmen employed in this part of the works

I 4   might

might suffer on account of their inad-
vertency. If the relation given by this
man was really true, it is great pity the
fraud was never difcovered, and a recovery of the metal attempted; as it
might eafily have been reftored by a little
trouble at the Finery, and made into a
better metal, either in the form of iron
or fteel, than before the accident happened. But to return:

With regard to the phyfical difference
between converted bar-fteel, and that
which hath been reduced from the bar
by fufion, it confifts principally in the
change, which is made by the different
arrangement of the atoms, which com-
pofe the metal; in the former cafe, after
it is taken out of the converting-furnace,
when broken, it ufually exhibits to the
eye,

eye, (if the iron made ufe of has been properly chofen,) the appearance of large fhining maffes; in the latter, there appears only a kind of a grofs grainy texture; with this effential difference between the two, owing to their different forms, that, though when they are reduced into rods, and their pores clofed by the hammer, and then properly hardened, when broken they fhall each of them difcover an equally fine grain; yet, fuffer them to be hammered into plates, or any flattifh inftruments, as razors for inftance, and when thefe are properly hardened and tempered, and after that finely polifhed, place them horizontally between your eye, and the light, and you will eafily difcover a very manifeft difference; for while the former fhall appear in this fituation, uneven and fcurfy,

I 5

no polifhed glafs can difcover a finer or
more even furface than the latter. Or, let
them be reduced into a proper form for
reflecting-mirrors, whether plane, concave
or convex, and treated as in the former
cafe, and the difference in their appearance
will exactly and uniformly correfpond to
the former inftance. I had the pleafure
of making feveral of thefe mirrors for
the very ingenious Dr. Ingenhouft, while
he was laft in England, which with fome
difficulty I found a method to get hardened, and then had them neatly polifhed,
much to the Doctor's fatisfaction.

But with regard to the uneven and
fcurfy appearance above-mentioned, I
apprehend that to be owing to fome
remaining quantity of foul fulphur not
thoroughly purged out, and hindering
the

the atoms from coming into proper contact; for let the bars of iron be hammered down with ever fo much care and
accuracy at the Chafery, and even after
they are converted into fteel, they will
yet be liable to many large blifters formed
on their furfaces, as well as in the interior parts, by the faid fulphur: but
when the bars of fteel are reduced by
fufion, the foul fulphur is fo far deftroyed
or driven out, that the atoms of the metal
are permitted to come into clofe contact,
and fo exhibit a fmooth uniform furface.

How thefe circumftances may affect
the edges of fine cutting inftruments, is
a matter of ftill farther enquiry. One
would naturally imagine, that while their
furfaces are liable to fuch irregularities,

I 6   it

it fhould be next to impoffible to preferve their edges entirely free from them.
Thus much I apprehend we may fafely
infer, that the fteel, which is remelted
from bars of converted iron, muft ftand
a much better chance to produce inftruments more pure, better connected in
their different parts, and confequently
not fo fubject to the above-mentioned
inconveniences, as when they are formed
directly from bars juft taken out from
the converting-furnace.

After all, there is ftill much more
knowledge and experience requifite, than
moft people are aware of, to produce fine
cutting inftruments, even though the method of reducing fteel by fufion has now
for fome years been known, and put in
practice.

I laft

I laſt ſummer took a journey to Sheffield, to try whether it might not be
poſſible to have the ſteel melted there,
upon ſuch terms, as to enable me to reduce the price of my razors, &c. but in
this I found myſelf greatly diſappointed;
for though I took with me ſteel of the
moſt excellent quality, converted for the
very purpoſe; though I prepared, and
carried with me, a ſufficient quantity of
my own flux, and had the ſteel melted
under my own immediate inſpection; I
ſay, notwithſtanding all theſe precautions,
when the ſteel came to be wrought into
razors, and other inſtruments, by one of
the ableſt artificers I could procure, they
fell ſo far ſhort of thoſe made from the
ſteel I had before melted, and wrought
down to proper ſizes, at my own manu-
factory,

factory *, that I could not honeſtly diſ-
poſe of them upon any terms.

Having

* The ſteel-manufactory in White-Croſs-Alley
in Middle Moorfields, where the beſt razors, lancets, &c. made by the author, may be had ; as alſo
at Mr. Thomas Wilkinſon's, at his warehouſe for
hardware, &c. No. 75. over-againſt St. Michael's
church in Cornhill. Were the author inclined to
ſacrifice to his own vanity, he might mention the
approbation and encouragement he hath received
from many great perſons, not excepting the greateſt
in the kingdom ; but he hopes to be excuſed in relating the following circumſtance, that when the
very ingenious Dr. Ingenhouſt was laſt in England,
after having been for ſome time in queſt of razors
peculiarly excellent, and almoſt every where diſappointed, he was by my late worthy friend Dr.
Gowen Knight furniſhed with my addreſs, and
ſending me a card, I took with me two dozen,
and left them with him for his choice upon trial.
After ſome time he informed me, he was quite
tired with trying the razors, as he could not find
one indifferent one amongſt them all: and accordingly he purchaſed at my own price the whole
number. It is with pleaſure I recollect the marks
I received afterwards of the Doctor's politeneſs and
friend-

Having said so much upon the first part of Mr. Reaumur's work, relative to his method of converting iron into steel;

friendship, and particularly, the several letters he honoured me with, when at Sheffield, containing a number of curious enquiries, as well as orders for various kinds of inftruments, which as I executed with pleafure, fo I had afterwards the pleafure to know, that it was to the perfect fatisfaction of my ingenious correfpondent.

It may not perhaps be amifs, if I take an opportunity in this place, of laying down a few rules for the management of razors ; and very few may fuffice.

After every operation, the razor fhould be gently applied to the ftrap, in the following manner :

The razor fhould be held in the hand in fuch a fituation as to prevent its turning on the rivet. This may eafily be effected by holding it at the fmall end of the fcale, in fuch a manner as to have fecure hold both of the fcale and the blade. Then let the razor be applied quite flat to the ftrap, fo as that the back and the edge may both reft upon the ftrap ; for if the blade be fuffered to form almoft the leaft angle with the ftrap, there will be

danger

fteel; I fhall, before I conclude, fubjoin
a few thoughts as to the latter part:
Entitled, *L'Art d'adoucir le Fer fondu,*

danger of turning the edge; which will for the
time render it utterly incapable of performing its
office. In this cafe the only method proper to
reftore it, is to draw the edge gently two or three
times over a little piece of horn, which generally is,
or ought to be, placed at the end of the ftrap.
This will deftroy, or break off this feather-edge,
as it is called: which is often performed by the
barbers by drawing it over the nail of their thumb.
Then give it a few ftrokes afrefh upon the ftrap,
which will certainly reftore it.

Many of my friends have affured me, that by
ftrictly adhering to the rules above-mentioned, they
have kept their razors in good order for feveral years,
without ever having occafion to ufe the hone. One
gentleman within thefe few days informed me, his
razor had been ufed for feven years, without
having ever touched the hone. Notwithftanding
which, I think it would be proper now and then
to have recourfe to the hone, as it certainly hath
a tendency, if it be done but gently and feldom,
to keep the edge of the inftrument in more compleat order.

The

The Art of nealing or foftening caft Iron ;
as to which however very little need be
faid, as I have reafon to apprehend, the
fuccefs in that attempt did by no means
anfwer his expectations; neverthelefs, to
fatisfy the curiofity of fome of my friends,
I fhall venture to lay before them what I
know of the matter, having tried in every
fhape the confequence of Mr. Reaumur's
doctrine. His reafoning is as follows:
viz. If impregnating with a fufficient
proportion of falt and fulphur will turn
iron into fteel; of a higher or lower
degree in proportion to the quantity
of materials proper for the purpofe,
which are made ufe of, and to the
time employed in the operation; then, if
I can find matter of a contrary nature,
which by being poffeffed of a fufficient
abforbing quality, will draw back and
drink

drink up the oppofite matter, by the ufe
of this you may rob the fteel entirely
of its fteely quality, and reinftate it in its
former condition, of being nothing but
fimple bar-iron. To afcertain the truth
of this hypothefis, he, as ufual, made ufe
of a variety of materials, and went through
a great number of experiments ; at length
he feems to have pitched upon calcined
bones of animals, reduced to powder, as
the bafis of his hopes of fuccefs in this
undertaking. It is well known that thefe
bone-afhes, as they are called, are the
matter made ufe of by the refiners, to
form their tefts, for refining their gold
and filver ; and as the medium employed
for that purpofe is lead, the quality of
which medium is to diffolve all the impure metal with which the pure metals
happen to be mixed, and to carry it off

in

in fume; that part of the impurity, which
is not thus carried off by fublimation, is
left to be abforbed by the bone-afhes
which form the teft. This confideration
was beyond difpute a proper foundation
on which Mr. Reaumur might expect to
erect his fuperftructure. But upon a farther profecution of the affair, he foon became convinced, that the material he had
pitched upon was not of a proper nature
to anfwer his purpofe; for though the
matter to be wrought upon, was not common fteel, but pig-metal; which it has
been obferved is fteel of the higheft degree, yet fo powerful was the material,
that at the fame time that it extracted
the falt and fulphur, it likewife by the
help of the fire neceffary to be made
ufe of in this operation, fo far calcined
the metal as to render it a mere crocus

of

of iron. In order to remedy this inconvenience, he was under a neceffity to
abridge and correct its power, by mixing
with it a certain proportion of charcoal
powdered; as follows, to two parts of
calcined bones, one part of powdered
charcoal. This mixture fo far anfwered
his purpofe as to reduce the metal. But
as his ultimate intention was to form fine
ornamental works from pig-iron, and then
after reduction by thefe materials, to have
them repaired and polifhed, here he mif-
carried; for though this method would
extract the fulphur and falt from the caft
iron, yet in producing this effect, it occafioned fuch a number of pin-holes, or
fmall vacuities on the furface, as rendered
his works utterly incapable of being
polifhed to any tolerable degree of accuracy.

I have

I have thus laid before my reader, a short
but faithful narrative of his whole scheme.
If any one should have an inclination, to
try any farther experiments upon this
bottom, he may safely pursue his design
from the hints here discovered, without
giving himself the trouble to peruse the
whole performance.

I have myself tried the truth of the
hypothesis in a rough way, as far as
nealing, or merely reducing, has any concern in the matter, by a great number of
experiments; two only of which I judge
necessary to recite by way of specimen.
I had several small ingots of cast iron,
about three quarters of an inch thick;
these I put into a crucible, covered all
round with the matter above described,
and in that situation committed them to
the fire, where I suffered them to remain

3   a suffi-

a fufficient time, then took them out, and gave them a ftrong heat; when the exterior parts were become capable of bearing even a welding-heat, while the interior fuffered an eafy diffolution, and ran out into the fire. I ran fome other ingots in the form of piftol-barrels, which having treated in the fame manner, the fame confequence enfued; the exterior cafes as before remained firm and ftable, while the interior, diffolved and ran out, and left cafes in the entire form of piftol-barrels.

And now on the whole, I think I have not made any material omiffion in the profecution of my defign; I only wifh the fubject had been treated with a greater degree of accuracy. To elegance of ftile I make no pretenfion; neither does the fubject require

quire it; embellishments of that kind are by no means requisite, where a faithful narrative of facts, founded upon cautious and well-tried experiments, is the principal thing in view. I may possibly be charged, and perhaps not altogether unjustly, with having here and there been guilty of tautology; all the apology I have to make, is, that the performance has been in a great measure compiled from old papers, written at different times; in reviewing which, in order to reduce the scattered hints into some resemblance of a regular system, it is next to impossible, that the same ideas should not sometimes have occurred again; and it might not be quite improper to repeat them, in order to impress them the more strongly on those persons, for whose benefit I am chiefly writing. Possibly I may be thought, in

3   some

fome few inftances, to have dealt too
freely with the character of the very celebrated Mr. Reaumur ; a character I extreamly revere, particularly as he was
the firft who attempted to reduce the affair of converting iron into fteel to a regular intelligible fcience. I wifh he had
been more fuccefsful in the attempt; but
he appears to me to have met with the
common fate which attends the under-
takings of all gentlemen in cafes of this
nature, who are obliged to place their
chief dependance upon fuch information
as they are able to collect from workmen,
many of whom are ignorant, and others
deceitful and impofing. Mr. Reaumur
himfelf very pertinently obferves the ignorance in this affair even of the great
Rohault, and intimates that he could
name an hundred others in the fame circumftance.

cumftance. And I have more than once had occafion to remark, in the courfe of this brief effay, how little dependance is to be had on moft of our lexicon, or dictionary writers, in fubjects of this nature; I venture again to offer it as my opinion that Dr. Harris, fo far as I may be thought a competent judge, greatly excels all his fucceffors in that way of writing; at leaft he deferves that character, in his judicious hints relative to the fubject before us. But it ought to be obferved, that Mr. Reaumur wrote his treatife in a great meafure to be an amufement for gentlemen, and the appearance of his book entitles it to a place in the genteeleft library; it is finely printed, the draughts contained in it are inimitably executed; but when you come to examine the vaft number of experiments he chooſes

K   to

to mention, I am greatly miſtaken, if
you do not find many of them extreamly
trifling, and of ſuch a kind that no rea-
ſoning, *a priori*, from the nature of the
ſubject he·was upon, could by any means
have led him into. And I do not remember to have met with a ſingle inſtance, where an artiſt in the ſteel-way
has ever profeſſed to have received
any·benefit from his writings. It is
now fifty years ſince his elaborate treatiſe made its appearance, during which
time, ſuch have been the improvements
in ſcience, particularly in magnetiſm,
electricity, &c. as has occaſioned ſtricter
enquiries into the nature of iron, and
ſteel, eſpecially the latter, ſo that gentlemen of education and ſcience are now
not ſo eaſily brought to ſit down ſatis-
fied with mere theoretic, and plauſible

7.   hypo-

hypothefes; but require fuch evidence as will ftand the teft of the ftricteft experimental fcrutiny. As I fet out with a profeffion, not barely to amufe this fort of fcientific readers, but likewife to free them from wrong preconceived opinions too haftily taken up, as well as to fecure them againft fuch mifapprehenfions for the future; I flatter myfelf I have not fallen very far fhort of my intention. However, I was at the fame time defirous, not only to approve myfelf to fuch gentlemen, by my endeavour to affift them in their laudable enquiries; but alfo to benefit thofe of my friends, and others, who are actually engaged in works of this nature, either in a more extenfive, or contracted way; and I hope this little performance will not prove without its ufe to them; as I am pretty certain there are

K 2   here

here and there a few hints to be met with, which have never occurred in any written accounts before; at leaft not in any one, that has ever fallen under my obferva-tion.

APPEN-

꧁꧂꧁꧂꧁꧂꧁꧂꧁꧂()꧁꧂꧁꧂꧁꧂꧁꧂꧁꧂

APPENDIX,

DISCOVERING

A more perfect Method of Charring
PIT-COAL, fo as to render it a
proper Succedaneum for Charred
WOOD-COAL.

꧁꧂꧁꧂꧁꧂꧁꧂꧁꧂()꧁꧂꧁꧂꧁꧂꧁꧂꧁꧂

K 3

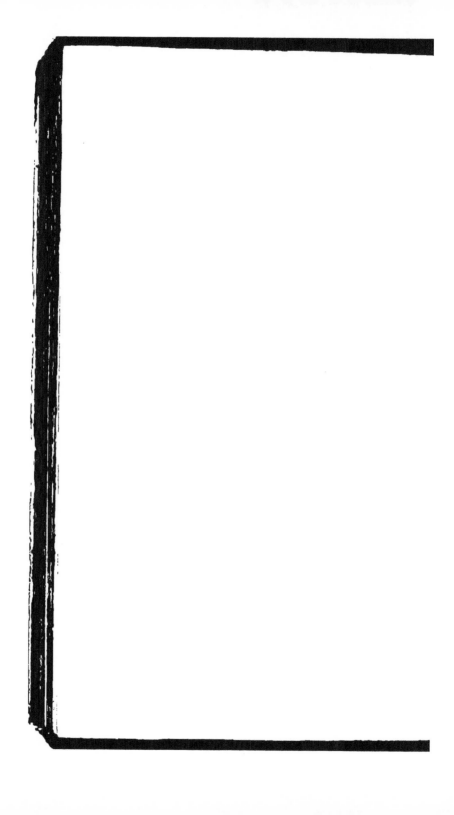

APPENDIX.

MANY attempts having been made to find out a proper method of reducing pit-coal, in such a manner as to render it a proper kind of fuel for the reduction of the iron-ore at the smelting-furnace, as well as for other operations afterwards at the other furnaces; and even at the various forges of the working cutlers, where a clean pure fire is always attended with peculiar advantages; and this matter still continuing a desideratum of the utmost consequence, I have made the accomplishment of it my particular study; and in the prosecution of it have spared neither pains nor expence.

As

As a foundation for this attempt, I found it neceſſary to be well aſcertained, what part of this uſeful mineral was requiſite to be diſcharged, as entirely noxious; and what part might be retained, as uſeful and ſalutary.

For this purpoſe, a few years ſince I ſpent ſeveral months at a friend's in Shropſhire, where I was informed ſeveral of theſe attempts had been made, and where at that time great quantities of this kind of fuel were made uſe of, in order to run down pots and kettles, as well as larger works, ſuch as cylinders for fire-engines, &c. Among other information which I was able to pick up in that part of the country, I met with a tradition that a famous Dutchman had made his appearance in that neigbourhood many years

ago,

ago, under the character of a great con-
noiſſeur in the ſmelting of iron-ore with
pit-coal: this perſon being thought to
have a conſiderable ſhare of knowledge
in this way, his propoſals were eagerly
embraced by ſome of the iron-maſters;
and no pecuniary aſſiſtance was refuſed
him, in order to put his ſcheme in exe-
cution. A very coſtly furnace was erected
for the purpoſe; much more ſo, than it
need to have been, had the projector
went upon true and genuine principles.
But unhappily, he had ſome how or
other imagined, that the flame iſſuing
from the fuel, becauſe it put on a clear
and ſplendid appearance, muſt be pure
enough, could it be conveyed to the ore
with ſufficient ſtrength, to be a proper
diſſolvent of it. To effect this, (as far as
I could procure any tolerable account of

K 5   the

the ftructure of the furnace, which for
many obvious reafons muft have been
a draught one,) the flame was by various
turnings and windings to have been fo
urged on, and directed by the force of
the air, as to terminate in ftrong and
powerful focufes againft the body of the
ore ; fo as to have procured a diffolution,
without any of the grofs parts of the
fuel coming in contact, or having any
immediate bufinefs in the operation.

Had the Dutchman better underftood
the nature of our mineral fuel, he would
never have fuppofed, that the flame could
by any means have furnifhed a pure or
proper diffolvent of the iron ore ; his
ignorance in this refpect defeated his project, as the metal feparated by this method difcovered fuch extreamly bad qualities,

lities, as rendered it abfolutely unfit, even for the moft ordinary purpofes. This ill fuccefs foon iffued in the breaking up of the fcheme, and the demolition of a very curioufly conftructed furnace.

Whether this mifcarriage furnifhed the firft hint, of the neceffity of charring the pit-coal, in order to render it ufeful, by carrying off the phlegm, and with it the more crude and hurtful part, of the raw and undigefted fulphur, I am unable to determine. But it is a fact now well known, that the method generally made ufe of for this purpofe, is burning the coal to a cinder, or turning it into what they call coke.

This operation is performed in various ways. Moft of what I faw burning for

K 6   this

this, and other purpofes, during my ftay for feveral months in Shropfhire, was performed in the following manner :

They raifed a pretty large circular hillock of raw coals upon the ground, covering them over with earth, only leaving a fmall paffage open, for the convenience of fetting fire to the heap ; and the whole heap being fet a burning pretty ftrongly, they then ftopped up the before-mentioned opening, with every other crevife they could poffibly difcover, to prevent any accefs of the common air ; which, however, fometimes, notwithftanding all their precaution, forced an entrance. Whenever that happened, the coals inftead of being burnt to a cinder, were reduced to a heap of afhes.

Such

Such a procefs anfwers the end extreamly well for the burning of peat,
where the afhes only are wanted, as a
valuable manure for land.

In the villages round about the me-
tropolis, where this fort of fuel is prepared for the ufe of the malfters, and fome
few other purpofes, they purfue a very different kind of management. They burn
the raw coals in ovens erected for the
purpofe, in fome convenient open place.
Thefe ovens being from time to time,
charged with a proper quantity of coals,
they fet them on fire. Near the front or
opening of thefe ovens the chimnies are
placed; at which outlets, when the coals
become fufficiently ignited, the flames,
which play round the interior parts of
the oven, make their exit, carrying along

7.   with

with them a very confiderable part of the crude fulphur.

It may not be amifs to obferve here, that the coals made ufe of for this pur-pofe at, or near London, are of a very different nature, from thofe which are dug up in Staffordfhire, Yorkfhire, and moft of the northern counties, which abound with mines of iron-ftone. The coals burnt about London, for making cinder, are generally, if not always, fuch as are brought from Newcaftle; which as they are not fo eafily reduced to afhes, but are apt, very frequently, to turn to obftinate vitrified clinkers, are by no means proper to be made ufe of for reducing iron in fmelting-furnaces, to form pig-metal, tho' they may ferve for fome inferior purpofes. But fuch coals only are fit to be made

ufe

ufe of for the above intention, as are
eafily confumed, leaving nothing behind
but pure clean white afhes.

But I fhould have obferved, that where
thefe ovens are made ufe of, the workmen employed at them, when they imagine
the coals are fufficiently burnt, draw them
out with an iron raker, upon the ground
before the oven, where they endeavour to
ftifle the yet remaining part of the fulphur, by quenching them with a deluge
of water. Thus they go on charging,
difcharging and fuffocating, till they have
compleated their intended quantity.

But as neither this method, nor that
which I had feen practifed in Staffordfhire, could upon the ftricteft experimental
fcrutiny be brought fully to anfwer the
wifhed-

wifhed-for purpofe ; I employed my ima-
·gination, to find out, if poffible, the effential reafon, why wood-coal charred fhould
effeđually anfwer fo many valuable purpofes, while pit-coal charred could fcarcely
be brought to any tolerable difpofition,
as a fuccedaneum, to anfwer fimilar in-
tentions. After having tried no inconfiderable number of experiments, and re-
volved the affair over and over, I at
length imagined at leaft, that I had hit
upon the true caufe.

I was fully perfuaded, with regard to
pit-coal, as well as wood or any other
materials fit for fuel, that after the more
hurtful, and corrofive part of the fulphur
was, in the fmoake and flame, fufficiently
carried off, if the remaining lefs noxious,
and lefs voracious fulphur, could be
brought

brought into a ftate as fixed and permanent
as that in the charcoal, I fhould become
poffeffed of the wifhed-for defideratum :
And the fixing of this remaining fulphur,
I apprehended, might be effected by the
burning coal being reverberated in a clofe
furnace or oven, till all motion fhould
ceafe, and the fire, as we exprefs it, go
out of itfelf.

At this time, a gentleman with whom
I was very intimate in Staffordfhire, informed me that there had lately been
difcovered in that neighbourhood a rich
vein of iron-ftone, from which great profit
had been expected; but that upon trial,
it had produced only a very bad kind of
red-fear iron; and that by attempting to
make ufe of it, in mixture with other
mine-ftone, it had communicated the fame
bad

bad quality to the whole mals. As I thought, that trying the effect of pit-coal charred according to the method I propofed, upon fome of this very bad mineftone, would, if it fucceeded, be reckoned a decifive proof of the utility and excellence of pit-coal fo charred, I acquainted my friend with my purpofe, and made him the following propofal: That if he would be at the expence of the materials, find a proper place, and employ an expert workman, to erect fuch an oven, as I fhould direct, I would take upon me the trouble and expence of fending down a fit perfon, to fee the whole executed, and the experiment properly made.

I fent down accordingly my own fervant, who had for many years accompanied me in all my experiments, one in whofe
judgment

judgment and fidelity I could place the utmoſt confidence; who having received full inſtructions, the building was properly erected, and made uſe of with all the ſucceſs that could be wiſhed for; a ſufficient quantity of the coal was prepared in it, which was left as above hinted to expire, and die away of itſelf, after the main part of the flame with the crude ſulphur had been conveyed up the chimney, and the mouth of the oven cloſely ſhut up and luted, to prevent any acceſs of the common air.

But before I proceed to enumerate the many advantages reſulting as the iſſue of this experiment, I apprehend it cannot be amiſs, to apprize thoſe of my readers whom it may more immediately concern, of ſome of the difficulties which occurred in the proſecution of it.

As

As I had been all along fuſpicious,
that the alternate elevation, and ſuppreſ-
ſion of the ſulphurous vapour, notwithſtanding ſo large a portion of it had been
carried off in form of flame, would of
neceſſity, when the mouth of the oven
came to be cloſely ſhut up, ſo as to prevent the leaſt acceſs of the external air,
or eſcape of the remaining ſulphur, occaſion ſuch an expanſion as might en-
danger the blowing up of the oven; for
this reaſon, I deſired my ſervant to take
all imaginable care in the conſtruction
of the oven, or furnace, and more eſpecially that the crown of it might be made
ſufficiently thick and ſtrong, capable of
reſiſting all oppoſition which might poſſibly be raiſed againſt it. In the courſe
of the operation all this precaution appeared to have been neceſſary; for notwithſtanding

withftanding thofe orders had been punc-
tually attended to, yet they were obliged
to lay a large additional weight upon the
crown, in order to be fully fecured againft
the apprehended danger.

This trial however, notwithftanding the
few difficulties that attended it, turned
out as fatisfactory as could have been
expected, or even defired. During my
fervant's ftay upon the fpot, he recom-
mended the trial of this fuel to feveral
ingenious artifts, and among the reft to
fome in the jewelling way, who were
hardy enough to make ufe of it in folder-
ing fome of their curious work ; for
which purpofe they declared it anfwered
the end as well as the beft charred wood-
coal they had ever met with.

Confidering

Confidering the matter as of great importance, I determined to make all the
experiments I could think of, in order to
afcertain the properties of this new fort
of fuel. I therefore procured a fufficient
quantity of the bad mine-ftone before
mentioned, and with it fome of the coke
or cinder, of both forts ; I mean fome
that had been prepared in the common
method of burning, and fome that had
been cured by burning in the oven I ordered to be erected for the purpofe.
Having roafted a quantity of the mine-
ftone, to render it fit for diffolution, I
put a part of it reduced to powder, into
a crucible, mixed up with a due proportion of the firft fort of coke, powdered
likewife, with fome of the common flux :
when this mixture came to feel a fufficient degree of heat from the fire, a feparation

paration was effected, without any extraordinary trouble; the operation, as I expected, produced a very bad red-fear kind
of iron, quite rotten, and of no value. After this I mixed up, in like manner, a fresh
parcel of the mine-stone, with some of the
coke that had been prepared according
to my direction; without any peculiar
degree of caution, except an absolute re-
jection of the minutest quantity of lime-
stone in the flux; instead of which I made
use of a very inoffensive flux, as cheap
and as easy to come at as lime-stone,
which I have sufficiently hinted at in the
foregoing essay. This reduction of the
same mine-stone turned out beyond my
most sanguine expectations. The metal
at the bottom of the crucible was so far
from being a red-fear rotten iron, that
in fact it was a very fine grained steel;

scarcely

ſcarcely malleable indeed, but ſuch as
with a proper degree of caution ſubmitted
to the ſtroke of the hammer, ſo far as to
bear beating out to a point, and afterwards underwent pretty kindly the pro-
ceſſes of being hardened and tempered.
In ſhort, the coke, managed in this method, I tried in every ſhape I could think
of, even for converting iron into ſteel;
and, in every inſtance, it appeared ſo apt
and proper a ſuccedaneum for charred
wood-coal, that, I own, I ſhould be at a
loſs which of the two to prefer for any
very curious purpoſe.

It may here poſſibly be enquired, how
ſo valuable a diſcovery came to be neglected, eſpecially in a part of the country
where ſo much buſineſs in the iron way
was carried on? This was owing to my
being

being in some sort connected here with two persons of very different qualifications; one an expert iron-master, the other only a country attorney, a little fond of dabbling in things which he did not well understand. Just when matters were ripe for excution, the former died; the other afterwards appearing to be a person, one would not wish to be concerned with, the affair was for that time laid aside.

It may likewise be objected, that an oven, or furnace, fit for the purpose, it should seem from what has been hinted, would be liable to many accidents and inconveniences; and that a great number of ovens would be requisite to supply a sufficient quantity of fuel for a large iron-work.

L   Thefe

These difficulties, I apprehend, are scarcely worthy of notice, provided the certainty of the doctrine laid down be well ascertained. The very first attempt, though attended with a few trifling difficulties, turned out in every respect so satisfactory, that there can be no doubt, a workman skilled in erections of this nature may be able to improve upon the scheme, by erecting such an oven, or ovens, as may be better adapted to answer the purpose, than that in which our first attempt was made.

As to the number which might be requisite to supply a large work, I would ask leave to interpose a query: Might not an oven be so contrived, as to have behind it, by way of reservoir, a vault sufficiently capacious to contain the quan-

3   tity

tity of fuel that might be prepared by fire, fix or more burnings in the oven? into which vault the fuel, when duly prepared, might be difcharged from time to time from the oven under fuch precautions, that when fo difcharged, the paffage from the oven to the vault might be ftopped. And as there muft of neceffity be an aperture fufficient to draw out the coke from the vault, that too muft be properly fecured againft accefs from the external air. But after all, no great difficulty or expence can attend the building of a fingle oven, in order to try the experiment: and if the operation be duly performed, according to the precautions laid down, I will venture to prophecy, that the event will exceed expectation, and certainly fupply a fuccedaneum, that will anfwer every purpofe

L 2   for

for which charred wood-coal can poffibly
be wanted.

After I had proceeded as far in this
operation as is above related, upon an
interview with my old fervant, he informed me, that it would be abfolutely
neceffary, in order to prevent the blowing
up of the furnace or oven, to leave fome
outlet in the top of the crown, that fome
part of the vapour might be fuffered to
make its efcape, when the expanfion happened to be too powerful for the building
to fuftain it : while, at the fame time, it
would be as neceffary to prevent fuch
efcape as much as poffible; fince the
greater the quantity of this fine fulphur,
which could be brought to a ftate of fixa-
tion, the better the fuel would be to
anfwer the purpofe. He was of opinion,
that

that this might be effected either by a proper valve, such as is made ufe of in the ſteam-engines ; or by ſome other ſimilar contrivance. As they had made no proviſion of this kind in the firſt furnace, of which he had the direction, they were ſubjected to great inconveniences ; for the ſtrength of the vapour ſeveral times forced its way through little breaches it had made in the building, which they were under a neceſſity of repairing in the beſt manner they could. As the ſtrength and force of the vapour declined, they took particular care to prevent any farther eſcape as much as poſſible, till at the latter part of the operation, they had brought their incloſure to form an abſolute occluſum.

After all theſe miſhaps and inconveniences, my ſervant aſſured me, that the fuel

fuel procured even in this imperfect manner, anfwered the purpofe, in all the trials
he had made of it, for reducing the mine-
ftone, much better than any charred
wood-coal he had ever made ufe of; for
he found the metallic atoms mixed in the
ftone, much eafier collected by it, and
likewife that it entirely prevented the
corrofive fulphur of the mine from cor-
roding his crucibles, which common charcoal would not always do. This laft-
mentioned advantage I cannot but look
upon as a very peculiar one, fince many
ufeful corollaries may, I think, be drawn
from it.

I have lately had it hinted to me by
a gentleman of good underftanding in
the nature of manufactures and commerce, as a thing much to be defired,
that

that this method of curing pit-coal might be rendered ferviceable to our wool-combers. I apprehend that this might eafily be effected; at leaft, the trial of it might be made at no great expence, as a fmall apparatus would be fufficient for that purpofe.

THE END.